The Writing
on the Wall

The Writing on the Wall

Regina Holliday

In Loving Memory of Frederick Allen Holliday II PhD

Table of Contents

Foreword To Regina Holliday's

The Writing On The Wall,

written by Mary Kay Zuravleff on March 31, 2015, Fred Holliday's birthday

REGINA HOLLIDAY IS A FIGHTER. Unfortunately, she's had more than her share to fight against. *The Writing on the Wall* is a manifesto for Regina's important advocacy work, her quest to unite technology with patient care.

Growing up in Sapulpa, Oklahoma, a town of scant prospects and few safety nets, Regina was determined to see the good in every situation. This kid could make a play kitchen inside a dank crawlspace; in a poor school in one of the poorest states, she looked forward to the outdated film strips on cell division as theatre. In fact, she used her imagination and artistic talent to survive childhood, as dire circumstances tried to squash her optimism at every turn. Regina managed to get not only through first grade, where she was daunted by dyslexia, but all the way to college, and though her father worked and beat her and her siblings, she eventually escaped from his sexual abuse to a shelter, saving her sister as well.

All those years living with a husband who was violent, mentally ill, and alcoholic, Regina's mother worked tirelessly. Regina still praises her tenacity: Bernice cleaned nursing home and hospital rooms, despite never getting insurance or having access to healthcare for herself. She even unwittingly cleaned up her own husband's trail of blood the night he was stabbed in a fight he started! Inspired by her daughter, Bernice finally extricated herself from her dangerous marriage, and so Regina probably saved her mother's life as well as her sister's. Her mother and her aunt, who was an intensive-care nurse, told Regina she should go into medicine. Regina recalled their wish when life dealt its cruelest blow yet.

But first, there were some good years. In a college painting class, Regina met Fred Holliday, and I met the two of them after they married and moved to Washington, D.C. We lived and worked in the same neighborhood, and after Fred's graduate school stint, they returned to the neighborhood with their son, soon followed by a baby brother.

My own rambunctious son loved crafts, and I often sought out Regina at the toy store because she had a million ideas. Theo was not looking for kits or sets; he wanted to create something grand, magical, or outrageous. Today, he is a furniture and tile designer, but at three years old, he was challenging. Regina knew exactly what the store had and how to use it; even better, she patiently encouraged him and offered clever approaches. Even when she couldn't satisfy him—there were no materials to help him make a flying car he could ride in—her attention and interest often did just that.

Regina's book is full of lessons she learned, and the lesson I learned from watching her is that listening to someone goes a long way, as does honoring their vision. She wanted to make a flying car, too—honestly, who wouldn't? Meanwhile, Fred worked next door at the movie-rental store, and we relied on his encyclopedic knowledge. My son loved raptors and didn't mind a vulture ripping apart carrion. But he hated movies where people were humiliated. Meanwhile, when we had a second child, a daughter, the age difference made for challenging choices. Fred steered us to some gems.

I write all this to give you an idea of the Washington, D.C., neighborhood we enjoyed. Like Regina, I also grew up in Oklahoma, and we have marveled at how this stretch of the nation's capital is like a small town only better. Our children walked to a good public school, where I was often room parent and Regina's talents were sought school-wide to help kids plan and make art projects. These class projects were sold at school auctions to pay for classroom aids, librarian, nurse, and other positions not covered by the DC Public School budget. Regina voluntarily painted murals inside the school, she helped organize the fall fair, and she was also the person who accepted donations next door to the school at the church's yard sale, which she headed. This woman helps people.

In the fall of 2008, Fred got his dream job teaching film studies and literature at American University in Washington, D. C. As it happened, I was hired that fall as American University's writer in residence, and we laughed at the coincidence when we saw each other at faculty orientation.

Fred loved his subject matter, and he hit his stride as a professor popular with both students and faculty members. Come spring, however, he could not shake the cold his family had passed around that winter. I remember his worrying that he was keeping Regina awake. In fact, he actually broke his ribs coughing, which should have led his doctor to do more than administer pain pills. While Regina and Fred took the boys to a pediatrician, neither was accustomed to being sick, pursuing healthcare for themselves, or demanding more attention than a doctor willingly gave.

It was Regina who pushed for the scans that revealed the cause of Fred's lingering cough. By the time her husband was diagnosed with advanced kidney cancer, he was already beyond a cure. Not that anyone told them that. Throughout Fred's short, horrible illness, Regina tried to get him humane care that fit his circumstances, as well as help for his formidable pain. She tried to get hospitals, doctors, surgeons, nurses, and physical therapists to answer her questions; she tried to minimize Fred's suffering. The two of them were educated, finally had health insurance, were valued at jobs they loved, and had strong community support. None of this altered the outcome.

What Fred went through was bad medicine practiced badly. He was subject to outrageous, nonsensical, and invasive procedures. When Regina realized how little time they had as a family, she was eager to make every moment count. But she had to spend their remaining days policing her husband's care—from getting him clean sheets to monitoring his meds—and fighting routines and decisions that caused Fred further agony.

Even during that ordeal, Regina was helping patients in similar circumstances. And on the day he died, she pledged to continue to be Fred's voice as well as your voice. That night, she posted her intentions on her blog, asking everyone to "do battle with me." Citing her mother's directive from years ago, she wrote: "My mother was a hospital housekeeper and my Aunt Minnie an ICU nurse. They always told me to go into medicine. Now, I will go *after* medicine."

In this poignant and devastatingly personal account, Regina likens the medical treatment she and her husband received to the abuse she endured as a child. Still optimistic, if you can believe it, ever-generous and incredibly talented, she works harder than anyone you've ever met solving her own and other people's problems. Just as she lived her childhood by her wits, imagination, and creativity, she is determined to affect change. She is using everything she has so you will get better treatment and be treated better in our medical community. She deserves our help and our gratitude.

Thank you, Regina, for this book and your efforts on this, what would have been Fred's forty-fifth birthday.

Introduction

WE COME INTO THIS WORLD red, screaming and owning nothing. We grow and change. The years pass by and we fill with life experience as our homes fill with possessions. Time rolls on and on, but for all of us there is an end. Some will meet their end on highways and some in hospitals, but for most of us the end is the same. We are patients in the end. We pluck at cloth hospital gowns, left with only a few possessions: our watches, rings and wallets.

A wallet says quite a bit about a person. It contains those few things we consider too important to leave behind. I have a very simple wallet and I love it dearly. I love its form because it reminds me of the many coin purses my mother used when I was a child. She needed a small purse to keep her coins for the snack machine at work. The purses were inexpensive and fell apart quickly; but they were well within the means of a poor child. I would buy them as a symbol of my love.

I also cherish my wallet because it reminds me of the staff of Newman Funeral Home in Grantsville, Maryland. They gave this wallet to me after my husband Fred's funeral. The wallet is a dark green and is emblazoned with a decorative panel and the words "Newman Funeral Homes." I didn't know funeral homes had promotional materials before Fred's death. I didn't know a lot about the process of dying. It's not something we talk about in our daily life.

Inside my wallet are some folded bills, identification cards and credit cards. Most importantly there are a few copies of my business card. I carry business cards everywhere. I hand them out on playgrounds. I hand them to fellow travelers on airplanes and at every conference I attend.

My business card has very little text. It simply states @ ReginaHolliday Artist, Speaker, and Writer. Then it lists my email address and my phone number. My card has very little text, but it is far from simple. Designed to look like a playing card, the Ace of Hearts to be exact, the business card is printed on a background as dark as the deepest night. The painting "Little Miss A-type Personality" appears on the center of the card. It is a painting of one of the darkest moments of my life.

Many people who look at my card remark on its beauty, I smile quietly and thank them. I wonder if they know that beauty and pain are often conjoined. Others chuckle and say, "Are aces high? Will you win the game?" Those comments remind me of the expression, "Life is a gamble." Sometimes you win and sometimes you lose; but it is so much harder to win when the deck is stacked against you.

Have you heard of ACES? It is the acronym for the Adverse Childhood Experience Study, a joint research project between Kaiser Permanente and the CDC (Centers for Disease Control and Prevention). It was conducted between 1995-1997 and the participants of this study are still being tracked today. Participants were asked if they had experienced adverse childhood events in their households, such as:

"Was a member of the family mentally ill or depressed?"
"Was a family member imprisoned?"
"Was your mother treated violently?"
"Was a family member an alcoholic or drug user?"

"Was a parent absent due to separation, divorce or death?"

Individuals in this study who answered yes to four or more of these questions were found to be at a substantially higher risk for chronic health problems and premature death.

The researchers of this study determined that children in the presence of abuse suffered adverse effects in their health. Just being in this hostile environment had a cumulative and toxic effect on the child. Children in the study who suffered four types of adverse experiences, it was determined that they were 260% more likely to suffer chronic obstructive pulmonary disease compared to a child without four adverse childhood experiences (ACEs).

To those who chuckled at my card and asked if I had won the game, the answer is yes. I am one of those lucky ones. I hold four of a kind in a game that no one wants to play. I am indeed lucky. I lived. I am a functional adult, I can maintain a job, and I carry my scars inside where very few people will ever see them.

When I first began to publicly advocate for needed change within the health care system, I rapidly learned there are things you do not say, things you do not do, and subjects you should not address. Audiences want to hear about solutions, bright spots and islands of excellence. Problems are fine to recount if they are quickly overcome by a new product, work management efficiency model, or leadership method.

You are not supposed to talk about God, you are not supposed cry, and you are not supposed to tell the world about abuse. My high school art teacher once told me, "You have to learn the rules, before you break them." This was the platitude that greeted my frustration at the endless quantity of soul-killing still-life drawings that I was forced to create in art class. I can proudly say I learned the rules of public health care advocacy and promptly broke them.

We have to talk about abuse if we are going to eradicate it. One of the most horrible effects of abuse is the destruction of trust that is needed for the creation of strong social networks. This is very sad because one of the best ways to advocate for yourself it is to tell your story far and wide. Since I began my advocacy, many of those who have heard me speak asked me if I would write a book. I said I would, but it would be different than many of the books that came before. Much of patient advocacy literature is focused on checklists, reference guides, and accounts of specific treatment scenarios. These "how-to" guides are vitally important during an encounter with the health care system, but they do not force culture change.

In the 1970s and early 1980s the public did not talk openly about child abuse. That changed when the faces of missing children appeared on milk cartons. People began talking about "stranger danger," and that opened up a door to a darker conversation. Strangers were not the only ones who could hurt you. I loved the faces on milk cartons because they empowered us all. Those faces appeared on the little pints we would drink at school. We, the children, read the question: "Have you seen this child?" We became part of the solution because we were asked to help.

"THIS IS NOT REALLY HAPPENING."
Often when I look at the institutional application of medicine, I see patients, families, and even staff suffering physical and mental abuse. Many families use some form of denial to live in an abusive relationship. They play pretend to everyone around them. "This is not that bad," they say. "We have a good medical system," say those who defend the current status quo. These individuals ignore the under-staffing, the unhygienic

practices, the inefficient paper work, and the lack of timely access to patient information at so many facilities. The staff and patients at such institutions are so mired in their day-to-day reality; they can see no other option of how to live than within their current cycle of abuse. An institutional system of care that does not protect its workforce from injury and leaves patients in the dark about the status of their disease is perpetrating great abuse within its walls.

"CHANGE WILL COST TOO MUCH."

I have known many women in my life who have stayed with abusive husbands because of money. "It will cost too much to leave him. He has the job. He could get the house and the kids." I always counsel people that the emotional cost is far greater. When a situation has become abusive it is your duty to take a stand. Now, as a nation we are making this choice. What harm shall we inflict to our national soul if we stand aside, and because of money, allow abuse to continue?

"WHY SHOULD THE GOVERNMENT MEDDLE IN MY BUSINESS?"

The government meddling is called regulation. Regulation can be a very good thing. It has lead to clear nutrition facts labeling, the clean air act, required seat belt use, and other amazing laws that save lives every day. We used to live in a world where it was okay to beat your spouse and kids. Go further back and it was okay to whip your servant. It is now against the law. The law of the land can change things for the better.

"IT WILL ONLY MAKE MATTERS WORSE IF I SAY ANYTHING."

We need immediate and real-time access to our medical record. We need this so we can speak out about what is going wrong and take ownership of our medical situation. We need patients to feel empowered to know that their thoughts are valid and they will not be penalized for speaking out. We need patients who will keep talking till someone listens to them.

The abused child will often have to report abuse to three adults before someone acts on his complaint. Patients and caregivers need to bravely step forward again and again to talk about the problems in the health care system.

"SOMETIMES IT IS NOT SO BAD."

Finally we come to the reason so many people stay in abusive relationships: there are the good days. There are moments of sunshine and light. There are hugs that are honest embraces not furtive gropes. In hospitals throughout our country, there are amazing dedicated kind people who are doing their best for their patients. There are providers who just go with the flow. There are uncaring and unsympathetic employees who make patients suffer.

We put up with the bad moments and bad people, because of the hope of getting better. We dread the belittling treatment of certain staff members while hoping the "nice" nurse is on duty today. It is a familiar quandary to a child of abuse. I write this book to tell you it is okay to say no. It is okay to say the current care situation is damaging and we must change it into something better.

Within my wallet is a business card. That business card may seem a simple a thing, but it contains my three-fold plea. I will paint about those who suffer, I will speak of those we lost, and I will write this book to convince you of the need for change. All I ask of you is to look, listen, and then act.

~Regina Holliday

Ending Where It Started

When I tell my children bedtime stories, I often finish with saying "the end." From personal experience, I think the phrase "the end" arises more from a parent's desperate desire to get some sleep than it does from a child's need for closure. I think even very young children reject the idea that a narrative exists only within the story. The three bears had many bowls of porridge before Goldilocks chanced upon their door. Cinderella cleaned many an ash pile before earning her name and walking on glass.

We happen upon characters while they are in the midst of their tale. Time is often compressed and decades are spanned within phrases. Sometimes the tales are of crisis and some are adventure or romance. The clock chimes midnight and time has stopped. The linear reality of our life falls away. These are the moments of fairy tales. Fairy tales are sometimes happy but are often quite dark. I find a medical crisis within a family feels very similar to the dark primal terror of the fairy tale. Like Alice in her rabbit hole, we are falling with no end in sight. When we finally reach bottom, do we drink the potion? Do we take the red pill or the blue pill? Sometimes for the story to move forward we must first remember what life was like when we were very small.

When I was young, my mother would tell me stories. Some of those stories were from my large nursery tales book and some of stories were read from Golden Books. I loved their compact shape and brightly colored pages. I would run my fingers over the shimmering gold on the spine of the book. I would beg my Mother to read it one more time. We did not buy many children's books; we could not afford them. But upon occasion, I would see the Golden Books display in the grocery store. I would plead with my Mother, "Please could we get one?" She would look down at me with her warm brown eyes and smile a half-smile. I would grasp the book with my pudgy hands filled with anticipation while standing bare-foot on the cool gritty linoleum floor. And she would say, "Yes." That night she would read to my sister and me and we would cuddle against her. Sometimes her stories were from the Bible. Sometimes she told us fairy tales. But I liked the stories of her own life most of all. I loved to hear her speak about her ten brothers and sisters growing up on a farm in rural Oklahoma. Some nights she would speak of her adventures in Colorado Springs when she was a waitress at the Stage Coach Inn. And rarely, for the bloom of love was fading, she would tell us of how she met our father and they fell in love.

My mother met my father in a hospital room. There are many patient advocates who expound the importance of the role of the caregiver; but I am one of the few who exist as a direct result of care giving.

My mother Bernice was a sweet girl who grew into a kind woman. She is second youngest in a family of eleven. Unmarried and in her thirties she had taken up the mantle of caregiver for her aging parents. Her mother Ella was small of stature; her legs bowed from years of hard work. Mom's father Reinhard was a tall man who still retained some of the vigor of his youth. He suffered from violent epilepsy so this caregiving task was a hard one. Mom lived with her parents in an old farmhouse in the country. Her social life revolved around farm tasks and church functions. She rarely spent much time in town before her father grew ill; but she stayed at my grandfather's side while he was hospitalized in Enid, Oklahoma.

My father had a troubled youth. As a child he was fond of hurting small animals. His relationship with his father was strained and his mother vacillated between bouts of despair and cloying affection. My father was dishonorably discharged from the Army due to his violent temper. He could never hold onto a job for very long. He most often worked at honkytonks and briefly owned a bar. He drank excessively and then would ride his motorcycle on the long lonely roads of Oklahoma. Dad had a horrible accident one night while riding with his current girlfriend. The girl died. My dad went to a hospital in Enid, Oklahoma.

Bernice was assisting her father Reinhard during his hospitalization in the 1960's. My father Gilmer McCanless was recovering in the shared room. They would share pleasantries and her care began to include both men. Slowly, amid white sheets and medicine their love began to bloom. I suppose some might say this was the Nightingale effect, for my mother was nothing like my father's prior loves. My mother was sweet and pious. Dad spent most of his time in beer joints and was prone to easy anger. But something grew between them in that hospital room; something that was once love and became heartbreak.

There are few moments in a life when everything aligns. In those moments we can make choices that will affect the rest of our life. Some call these moments providence. Regardless of what we call them, such a moment occurred between my parents. My parents should have never met. They both had very different views on God and politics. They lived in very different social worlds. But in the 1960s, shared hospital rooms were the norm.

My father could be charming and perhaps he charmed his way into my mother's life. Or perhaps he was hurting and she was there. Regardless of whatever transpired during those days of care giving, the result was marriage. My father loved my mother and my mother loved him back. In the years that would follow when things became so dark,

I would question that love. Did he ever truly love her? Did he love any of us? Then I would think of the image seen within a broken mirror. A shattered mirror still reflects an image. It is just a distorted image. My father was a very broken man and we were his reflection.

Mother was a good caregiver. She did her best to love and cherish each of her children within the confines of a bad marriage. She would teach me those skills to apply within my life. In school, I would often befriend those who suffered more than myself. During my brief time in the Navy the other recruits would call me Momma McCanless due to my care giving ways. Then I married Fred and a lifetime of care giving stretched before me. Fred was funny and vivacious, but also suffered from anxiety and depression. Many a time Fred would wake me up at 3:00 in the morning. He would be in a panic about a paper that was not going well, or he would worry about a test. Regardless of the challenges in our life, we would face them together and we would care for each other.

So if the story of my life has a beginning, it started with care giving in a hospital room; and my life, as I knew it, ended many years later in another hospital room. At the age of 37, I was the caregiver. My husband was the patient and he was slowly dying. Then I would understand what my mother must have once felt. For the love you feel as a caregiver can melt the heart of the hardest of men. That same love can break the heart of the kindest of men as well.

Holding On And Letting Go

In the summer of 1976, I was four years old.

This was the summer when every coffee tin in the grocery store isle was adorned with a flag. This was the summer that my mother bought her commemorative liberty bell cookie jar. This was the summer Americans were told to go on the road and rediscover our proud country. Our family followed this national tide of travelers and began a road trip that would take us from Oklahoma to Kansas, Missouri, Nebraska, Colorado, and New Mexico. It was a magical time. We piled into our brand new '76 Chevy Impala and tasted the freedom of the road. Even though I was only four at the time, the experiences of those Kodachrome brilliant summer days are seared within my mind.

While in Colorado we visited an amusement park called Santa's Workshop. Ten miles west of Colorado Springs, there was a North Pole experience complete with a candy cane slide. It felt very odd to run from activity to activity in the warm sunshine while surrounded by buildings adorned with painted snow. The amusement park also claimed to have the tallest ferris wheel in the world. I will never forget the moment I rode that wheel. My family peered up at the huge ferris wheel built upon a mountain at an altitude of 7,500 feet. The operator dared us to ride the enormous structure. My mother chuckled and said she would not. My father laughed as well. My brother and sister stepped back.

I stepped forward.

The man asked if I was sure. Did I really want to ride all by myself? I nodded yes, and was lifted up into the seat. The operator pulled down the restraining bar and locked it into place. That bar floated a good eight inches above my legs. I looked at the other carriages and found I was one of very few people who had attempted the ride. As my seat rose ever higher, my knuckles whitened around the restraining bar. I realized how easily I could fall. I looked at the great space between my legs and the bar. I stared at my little fingers pressed so tightly on the cool metal bar slightly eroded by rust. I looked down at my scuffed canvas shoes as they dangled so many feet above the crowds. As I reached the pinnacle of the ascent, I looked far below at my small family.

At that moment, I felt so proud, so strong; I alone had braved the ride. I was filled with fear, but I would not let it panic or conquer me. I was so glad that I got to do this. I cherished the moment and the trust my parents had in me. Even though I was only four, I could be brave. I was joyous and I was on top of the world. It was a wonderful vacation. We were happy for the most part

My mother had just gotten her inheritance after her father's death. We had a new car. Dad put a down payment on a Mac truck and told mom he would become a truck driver. We purchased a brand new mobile home. Mom always called it a mobile home, but I supposed you could call it a trailer since we moved into a trailer park.

I was five years old by the time we moved. I loved the newness of our house on wheels. I loved the bunk beds that were purchased for my sister Esther and me. Life was mostly good. I even tolerated my older brother Eugene. I more than tolerated his friend Robbie; I fell in love with him. He was much older than I and at ten years of age way out of my league. Even though I was just a little girl, sometimes the big boys would let me tag along in their play.

Culverts and ravines surrounded our trailer park outside of Tulsa. It was a perfect landscape to play war. Robbie and my brother were often soldiers, and I was a *M.A.S.H* nurse who carried a toy AK-47. I remember one truly epic battle when Robbie was "shot" by the enemy. He fell to the ground moaning with all the dramatic anguish that a ten-year-old boy could muster. I knew I had to move him toward a culvert and out of the line of fire, so I dragged him few feet and saved Robbie from the *war*. But I think my brother Eugene got jealous of the time I spent with Robbie, not long after that incident he told me about mushrooms.

Mushrooms often grew in our yard. I was inspecting a mushroom by touching its cool pliant surface, when Eugene yelled out behind me, "Don't touch that!" I quickly pulled away and put my hands behind my back. He looked at me sternly and asked if I had touched the mushroom. I lied and told him I had not. He breathed a sigh of relief, and said, "Good! Those are poisonous and just one touch would kill you by bedtime." Then he walked away.

I must admit I was rather scared. But how many days from our childhood do we remember with crystal clarity? I truly enjoyed that day I was going to die. I played with abandon. I was very kind to my little sister and bequeathed her all of my toys. I had fried chicken with mashed potatoes that night for supper and relished watching *The Incredible Hulk* on TV. Everything smelled so wonderful, colors were so bright, and people were so good. I put on my favorite nightgown that night. I snuggled into my bed divested of all my worldly possessions. I said my prayers with my mother and sister. When my mother said goodnight, I said goodbye.

That is when the proverbial you-know-what hit the fan.

My brother was in big trouble. Those mushrooms were not poisonous. He still giggles about that story, even into his late 40's. But I thank my brother, because I still have a crystal clear memory of a day from my childhood. I thought I was going to die, and I made peace with that. He meant to play a trick on me, but instead he gave me a most precious gift.

Later that same year, I wore my favorite nightgown again. I spun in circles like a ballerina. It was such a pretty gown; it was long and tiered with lace. It would balloon around me as I spun, and I felt so beautiful in that gown. After a final spin, I smiled at my mother and said, "I love this gown so much I want to be buried in it." She looked at me with disapproval and said, "Hush, don't say such things." I was very confused. I thought, why wouldn't my mother want to know my wishes if I died?

As I write these words, I live many miles from Oklahoma in a small town in Western Maryland. I try to visit my mother each summer. She is getting on in years. She used to laugh on her birthday and tell us she was "39, just like Jack Benny." I would tell her casually referencing Jack Benny places her a lot closer to eighty than forty.

Mom has trouble moving around these days and wanted my help to go through her closet during my last trip. We packed up two large bags of clothes for charity. Then she picked out a favorite dress to remain in the closet and asked me to write a sign for it. "Bury me in this," says the simple note. I understood those sentiments exactly, and in my memories a little girl in a nightgown spins in circles of joy.

Things Fall Apart, The Center Cannot Hold

"Trailer for sale or rent,
Rooms to let fifty cents.
No phone, no pool, no pets;
I ain't got no cigarettes.
Ah, but two hours of pushin' broom
buys an eight by twelve four bit room.
I'm a man of means, by no means king of the road."

BY ~ROGER MILLER

THAT SONG ALWAYS REMINDS ME of my father. I think of his whiskey-soaked baritone with its hint of an Oklahoma twang. He had the type of voice that some singers aspire to. I always wondered why anyone would want a whiskey-soaked voice; whiskey is dangerous. The song reminds me of him not only because of its timbre and tone. This song could be his anthem.

By 1977 my father gave up on being a truck driver. He could not keep up the payments on the truck and the creditors took it away. My mother had a bout of Bell's palsy. She had to wear an eye patch and she stopped smiling due to her crooked face. As our family income dwindled, the mobile home proved itself true to its moniker. The trailer and the entire family moved to Enid, Oklahoma. We had relatives in Enid, so I looked forward to moving there.

I loved to visit Aunt Minnie and Aunt Hilda. They had houses across the street from each other on a quiet cul-de-sac. They were kind and always had good things to eat. Aunt Hilda was the spinster aunt, having never married. She dedicated her life to God and her work at Gold Spot Dairy. She was the stern one, the one who did not let things pass. She corrected behaviors frequently and therefore any praise that came from her lips was doubly sweet. She was an excellent cook and made my favorite desserts whenever we would visit. I especially enjoyed her rice pudding. She smiled the most beautiful smile and her joyful laugh would echo around a room.

Aunt Minnie's house always smelled of flowers and cinnamon. Aunt Minnie was a widow; she nursed her husband for many years before he died. She was my jolly Aunt. Throughout my childhood, her refrigerator was covered with magnets from her nursing career, her Lutheran faith, and one chubby wooden sheep that said, "ewe's not fat, ewe's fluffy!" The ceiling was ringed with a set of commemorative dishes from *Little House on the Prairie*. In the corner was a macramé plant holder made by one of my cousins so many years ago. The kitchen did not change in all the years she lived there; each Christmas she would just add one more layer of homemade gifts from our far-flung family. Aunt Minnie would sit upon her recliner watching game shows and soaps. Her corded phone was extra long to stretch over to her beloved chair. That was important because Aunt Minnie kept 100 plus family members and many friends connected through her calls. Aunt Minnie was a nurse in an Intensive Care Unit at St. Mary's Hospital in Enid, Oklahoma for many years. She worked the 3 pm to 11 pm shift. I remember being small and visiting her at Christmas. She would eat the family meal with us then dress in her uniform and go to work. I thought it unfair, but she said the patients especially needed nurses on Christmas.

We children enjoyed our time in Enid. We loved visiting family on a regular basis, but Dad could not find a job he was able to keep. Bills began to mount up and soon my parents could not make payments on the mobile home. We would have to move again. My father drove the moving truck filled with our possessions. Mother gathered my brother, sister and me into the Impala, and we drove to Sapulpa, Oklahoma.

My paternal grandfather Raymond McCanless lived in Sapulpa. We children called him Krackaw. My eldest cousin Sandra gave him that name when she was just a toddler, as she could not pronounce the word "Grandpa." I loved Krackaw. He had false teeth that he would move in and out of his mouth while he danced a jig wearing cowboy boots. We had lived with him before. He had taken us in when money was tight. He owned an old house on Elm Street three blocks from downtown and the county courthouse. Sometimes I would walk downtown with Krackaw. He would walk slowly in his cowboy boots and spit chaw into the weeds beside the path. He would tell me tales of long ago. I would scamper beside him like a puppy, my bare feet skimming the pavement as I circled around him. We would visit Rexall's Drug and he would buy me a soda pop in a glass bottle. I would relish the cold drink and trace my finger upon the beads of perspiration on the glass. I would wait patiently as he joked with the shop-keep or flirted with the ladies at the till. One day near the register, I noticed this blue-lettered chipboard sign covered with little red paper flowers. I asked grandpa if I could have one of the flowers. He purchased it for me and as I admired it in all of its crepe paper glory, he told me, "Someone died for that." I looked up at my grandpa in confusion. He opened the door and ambled down the path with his loose-fitting boots clopping upon the pavement and continued. "I was born in 1907. When I was a boy there was a war and many soldiers died. After that war, they started making them poppies. Everyone of them poppies is a dead person."

Krackaw would often tell me such stories. He was full of stories. He would tell me of the time they disassembled a neighbor's model-T Ford and resembled it on the man's garage roof as a Halloween prank. He told me dandelions were evil plants. I would watch Krackaw walk endlessly in our back yard with his dandelion pruning fork. He would move from flower to flower lopping off the blossoms in an endless futile battle. It was futile in part because every flower he missed would develop a beautiful puff of seeds. My sister and I could not help but make a wish and blow them all over our yard. Even without our dubious help he was bound to fail. Dandelions are not only great at spreading their seeds, they have a taproot that is ten inches long. If any of the roots remain in the ground, the plant will continue to grow. Krackaw has been gone for many years. His house where I grew up was leveled. But when I visit that empty lot, I am greeted by dandelions.

Krackaw's house had three bedrooms and a nice big yard. The house was covered with lovely green and white striped asbestos siding. The windows were overhung with quaint sheet metal awnings. The house was on a double lot and surrounded by a five-foot high wire fence. In spring and summer the fence became a hedge of flowers. There were honey suckle, morning glories, and trumpet vines. In the center of the back yard stood a native Oklahoma pecan tree well over 80 feet tall. Each year we would harvest the sweet hard-shell nuts that fell in abundance from the tree. Beside the tree, Krackaw and my father had built a children's playhouse. I did not know it then, but we would live in Krackaw's house for the rest of my childhood.

When I was a small child we would also walk around Sapulpa with our mother. I remember trips to the grocery store. Esther and I would each carry something small in our pudgy hands as my mother struggled with the paper bag filled with groceries. We would scamper with her to the post office. It was a grand and honorable place with marble columns and brass trimmed service windows. As we would enter the monumental building with its magnificent foyer, I would marvel at the spacious height of the ceiling. My footsteps would echo upon the speckled marble floor and I would wait in silent awe as we stood in line to mail a package or buy a sheet of stamps. My mother would open her coin purse and count her coins and dollars. The mail clerk would hand her a glassine envelope filled with stamps. I would stare at that envelope seeing the distinctive dips and swells of the gummed paper edges of the stamps contained therein.

If I were very good, when we returned home I would get to lick the stamps and place them upon the letters. I would taste the unusual flavor that only comes from gummed paper. Then I would proudly place those letters in the mailbox. Sometimes I would wait upon our porch as the cicadas hummed their summer song and wait for the mailman to take the letters far away.

Although, the small town of Sapulpa was a great place to raise a child, there were not many jobs available for someone like my father. So this time he did not even try to get a traditional job. He decided to become a junkman. As the years passed by, my grandfather's pretty lawn would fill with pile after pile of broken furniture, old metal tools, fiberglass storage canisters, and box after box of *treasures*. My father would sort through the endless detritus, select enough to fill a pickup truck, and spend all day Saturday and most of Sunday at the Sapulpa Flea Market. He had finally had found his calling. He was finally his own boss. No one could fire him no matter how badly he behaved. He even had three small children for employees.

I have worked many jobs in my life and have always been commended for having an excellent work ethic. I was taught the value of hard work at the age of 6 with a limber switch. I was taught to never socialize with my fellow workers by a man who used words that cut like knives. In the bitter wind or oppressive heat, I would stand on a concrete slab and sell junk all weekend. If we behaved well and sales were good, our father would pay us each two dollars. The remainder he would take and spend on beer.

Needless to say, our mother had to get a job or we wouldn't have anything to eat. She only had an eighth-grade education so her choices were slim. The nursing home in town was always hiring, so in her late 40's she began to work at the backbreaking task of cleaning every day. They were understaffed and undersupplied so my mother's job was a hard one. Mom's co-workers came and went like the flies that buzzed around the mouths of the residents. She did her best to help the elderly denizens. At Christmas she would have Esther and me dress in our best dresses and sing carols for the lonely residents who had no family of their own.

When our family moved back to Sapulpa, I struggled in school. I had just finished a year of kindergarten in two different school systems. My mother tried to help me understand my lessons. She didn't like to write very much herself, although she had excellent penmanship. She often laughed after making a statement. As though to say, "If I didn't say that right, it was only a joke." (I tend to do this too, especially if I am nervous.) She has the sweetest crooked smile that resulted from her case of Bell's palsy. I remember the eye patch she wore as she helped me with my homework. I was trying to learn my letters. I had written them all backward. She held the sheet up to a light and turned it around and said, "See, that is the way it is supposed to look."

First grade was a blurry lack of understanding. I remember my complete confusion about the purpose of letters and numbers. I could not understand what the teachers wanted. The teacher told me A was for apple. Great, I get it. A=Apple. No, that was wrong. She tried to explain phonics to me, and I didn't comprehend. Fine! I could not read nor write, but I could draw. I came up with a brilliant plan; I would draw an apple and then she would understand. That plan didn't work. On the last day of school my teacher gave me a card with a picture of bees buzzing by. When I got home my mother read the note to me. It said I would have to return and repeat first grade. "I would bee back."

I had flunked. My few friends were now in a second grade. My little sister Esther had now aged into my grade. She was doing so well in school. Her penmanship was perfect. She kept clothes very nice and did not play rough sports with the boys, as I was wont to do. I think she was somewhat embarrassed by her older sister.

During the second year of first grade, my class was held in the overflow classroom in the basement of the school, beside a storage closet. It was one of very few classrooms at that level. It was dank and smelled of must and mold. I could not help but feel this was some kind of punishment. At mid year our room was vandalized. The vandals poured endless ribbons of our school glue throughout the room. For the rest of the year, the chalkboard was challenging to use due to all the raised lines from the adhesive. I still did not really understand reading and math. I would draw elaborate pictures as my teacher spoke. Perhaps if I could draw the lesson, she would be pleased. She was not. She sent me to the principal's office. The principal was often gone, so the secretary would hand me crayons and paper and I would spend the time away from my class drawing.

Each day at recess, I would immediately run to the far corner of the playground. I would pick up the pieces of Oklahoma sand stone and methodically rub them against the concrete wall. At first, they were an inexpensive chalk and I would draw images. As I rubbed longer, I realized I could sculpt the stones by rubbing them. I made primitive carvings this way. When I watched Stephen King's *The Shawshank Redemption* in 1994, I thought of the seven-year old me trying desperately to stave off the loneliness and feelings of imprisonment by carving stones like a little Andy Dufresne. Stone carving takes a long time. It is an art form adopted by those who measure time in weeks and days not minutes or hours.

As if school was not enough anguish, my father was torturing me at home. With words and belts and switches, he was making every day a private hell. I wondered what I had done wrong to suffer so. It is hard to be seven years old and wonder if today was the day I was going to die. We had a print of Pablo Picasso's *Guernica* on our dining room wall. The print was approximately 2 1/2 feet by 5 feet. I would eat my Frosted Flakes cereal and study anguish. Have you ever stared at *Guernica*? There are dead babies in that painting. I vividly remember being beaten by my father and staring at that painting on the wall through a sheen of tears. While the welts rose on my legs and the switch danced through the air, I saw a kind of compassion in the piece. It was a sense of shared suffering. If I could just draw, God would deliver me.

In The Dark Of Play

WHEN I WAS A CHILD, the summers were hot and the basement was cool.

Some days the mercury would rise to 115 degrees. I would look into our backyard and across the alley. Above the asphalt parking lot behind our house the air would ripple like smears of grease on a television screen.

Inside it was sweltering and fans whirled in some vague attempt at cooling the seven rooms of our house. There was one window unit air conditioner fighting a losing battle in the dining room. The unit rattled and you could keep cool if you stood right in front of it. I often thought the air conditioner was most appreciated by the patch of green moss that lived outside. The moss was fed by the continual drip of water droplets from the condenser coil.

There was a cool basement below us. Perhaps I should call it a cellar rather than a basement. Some of our friends had basements with upright interior entrance doors. Those doors led to descending staircases well lit with electric light. Such basements were often the playroom or family room. They were carpeted even if they occasionally smelled of damp.

Our basement had a sloping exterior door and looked like a storm cellar. At the age of eight, I could barely open the heavy door if I strained with all my might. When opened, strands of spider's web would waft in the breeze as a rush of cool, musty air arose from the open door. Each step down was made upon aging concrete. My small body would step deeper into darkness surrounded by cellar walls consisting of a mismatch of sandstone and brick. At the base of the stairs the light from the sun lit a five-foot area.

As I descended into darkness, I would need to duck beneath the trailing spider webs. Then, eyes blinded by the bright outside sun, I would shuffle barefoot across the gritty cool floor toward the dangling chain of the incandescent light.

I would wave my hand in front me feeling for the metal ball chain and gratefully pull it. Snap. The light came on and a dull amber glow filled the dank space. The basement was bi-level. Within our rectangular basement an L shaped area was somewhat finished with a concrete floor and a sump pump drain. The sump pump hummed within its inky darkness and the floor around it was wet. The area of the basement that was not part of the L was a raised earthen embankment two and half feet above the floor.

The walls of the embankment were concrete and were edged with supporting pillars for the house above. These pillars were made of sandstone, old bricks from the brick plant, and steel pipes. I would heft myself upon the raised embankment and crawl between the pillars to a little play kitchen I had created along the back wall. Here was a small basement window, but I pretended it was the kitchen window. The dirty glass let some light into the space. I had taken a few pieces of rusted iron parts and had fashioned *burners* on my sandstone stove. There I would *cook* with my toy dishes and picnic with my dolls in a room that smelled of the grave.

Have you ever crawled in the cool dirt of an unfinished basement? There is a musty earthiness, a quiet stillness. Every once in awhile a ray of light from the small window would alight upon a rock and I would see the mineral sparkle of the stone.

I would see the sparkle in the darkness.

There were spiders down there in the basement. Hundreds of brown recluse spiders surrounded me while I played. There was mold and damp and darkness, yet I will never forget the sparkles of the stones in a shaft of light or the wonder of play. I knew even then that you could make something out of darkness.

Often I would play alone in the basement. Sometimes my sister Esther would play with me. She was slight and small with large velvet brown eyes. Esther loved dresses with lace and sometimes wished the world were made of pink. Yet she still would play with me in the darkness. For moments we were happy among the trailing webs and the musty dirt. We knew there were far worse things than spiders in the dark. Upstairs was where the real monster lurked.

Upstairs the walls could weep.

Each night I would watch the droplets roll slowly down the walls of my bedroom. My mother explained the walls lacked insulation, but I knew it was more than that. The cool night air would embrace a room filled with the warm breath of two little girls; then it would cry for us. Each tear track left its mark and the lower walls were covered with black mildew variegation.

These walls had suffered much. Here and there were the telltale signs of violence. The drywall had holes shaped like fists and indentions from steel toe work boots. Scrawled upon the wall were words. These were not the crayon musings of a child. No, these were dark words written with permanent marker, a mixture of uneven capitals and the occasional cursive lower case letter. "No FooD or DrINK in THis rooM" or you will be punished.

Even in this darkness there was some light. Two embroidered prayers hung with honor on these walls. My mother had sewn a morning prayer and an evening prayer. These pieces were my mother's art. Little embroidered bunnies scampered upon the cloth next to my mother's neatly spaced letters in a reassuring font. My sister Esther's prayer was the morning one and it began with: "The sky is blue the sun is bright, the Lord has kept me safe all night." The prayer suited my little sister and her life to come.

I loved my evening prayer and reassurance that if I should die before I wake, the Lord would take me far, far away from fists, boots and walls that weep. So within this room of my childhood were the portents of my future advocacy. Here I would lay awake at night and think about suffering and death. Here I would look at the writing on a wall and realize words placed where they do not belong can be hard to ignore.

Chickens And Kittens

A BARGAIN IS A TRICKSY thing. My father Gilmer loved his bargains. As a junk dealer he often bought items by the box lot. We children would sort out his mysterious treasures. As an adult I often sift though data in an endless stream. My friends and fellow advocates sometimes ask, "How do you manage following so many different conversations?" They would not wonder at my sorting ability if they could only see my childhood.

There was the summer we sorted nails. My older brother Eugene, Esther and I stood in the glaring Oklahoma sun. The locusts droned their summer chorus as we three looked at the expanse of rusty nails, screws, and bolts before us. We stood around a wooden tray four feet wide and six feet long. It contained an iron wasteland of nails and screws three inches deep. We were supposed to sort all of these fasteners by type into small baby food jars. Our fingers turned orange with rust and our faces dripped with sweat. We were not supposed to talk with each other. I tried to sing to help my mind escape the heat and the onerous task. Dad yelled out from the shade tree from where he sat with his beer bottle, "No singing." I thought that was not fair as even slaves were allowed to sing. In my mind Dad corrected me with his mantra, "Life's not fair."

Next we sorted shoes. Dad had purchased a truck bed full of un-matched pairs for a great price. Our back yard was filled with row upon row of shoes each looking for its partner. Years later when I visited the shoe room in the Holocaust Museum in DC, I would be reminded of the summer of the shoes. Some shoes smelled of mildew and were dusted with a green powder of mold. Those we would clean with rags. The nicer shoes Dad would have us polish. We spent broiling days working on the shoes. Then Dad would sell them for a quarter a pair at the local flea market and drink the proceeds.

But bargains were not limited to the things we sold; bargains applied to the things we ate as well. Once Dad purchased a five-gallon drum of lime green Jell-O at an absurdly low price. We had to eat lime green Jell-O for years. Decades later as my husband Fred was sick in the hospital I would stare in disgust at the green transparent square that jiggled on his hospital tray. To this day I despise lime green Jell-O.

But the bargain of chickens was far worse than Jell-O. As a poor family we always struggled to make our food budget stretch. Dad would yell at Mom when we would have meals without meat. "A man is supposed get meat at a meal!" he would yell. She tried, but on the salary of a housekeeper she just could not afford the high price of meat. So mostly we ate macaroni or fried potatoes. Fortunately, our family lived with our Grandpa and he received government cheese because of his social security benefits. I loved that government cheese. We had a lot of grilled cheese sandwiches. We would finally get meat on payday. Mom would make hamburgers or occasionally chicken.

Then one day Dad came through the door smiling, which was rarely a good thing. He said "I just got the best bargain on chicken." Mom asked where he was shopping. He replied on the side of the road. He led us out to the covered bed of his pickup truck. In the bed of the truck were five chickens and a rooster. They were very much alive. It was illegal to have live chickens within the town limits, so Dad put them all down in the basement. It was a horrible time. The rooster did not know day from night within the darkness. The rooster would crow at all hours. Dad said not to worry because we would kill the rooster soon.

My mother grew up on a farm and knew how to kill a chicken, pluck it and clean it. My rational mind knew that chickens die everyday on farms throughout the country, but I thought very few of those chickens spend their last days trapped in a dark basement before the slaughter. It troubled me that Dad was able to hide the rooster from the neighbors, that no one would hear its cries, and then he would simply kill it.

On the day we were going to slaughter the first chicken, our friends, fraternal twins Katie and Angie, came to watch. We were town kids so none of us had ever seen something like this before. As we waited for the process to begin, my mother asked me to take out the trash. I dragged the large trash bag towards the alley. Then I saw a man in a pickup truck dump a bag on top of our trash. I walked closer to our old tin trashcan and saw the bag *move*. I dropped my bag and ran to tell Esther and the twins. We all ran back to the alley. We carefully opened the sack and eyes stared back at us.

There were four small kittens in the bag. We scooped them up and held them with loving caresses in response to their quiet mews and scratchy tongues. We ran to Mom and Dad and showed them off proudly. We asked why they were left in a bag in the trash. Dad responded while he was sharpening the axe, "That shit for brains who dumped them should to have wrung their necks first before putting them in a trash can." He then placed the axe on the wooden stump before him.

We begged Mom and Dad to keep the cats. We had never had pets before. Dad told the twins that they could take whichever ones they wanted, but he told Esther and me that this was a real responsibility. He looked over to us and said, "I will make a bargain. If you girls keep those cats you have to feed 'em and care for 'em. They never get to live in the house. And if you don't care for them I will chop those pussies heads off just like this here chicken." *Thwack!* With that said, the axe went down. I then learned there is a reason for that phrase *"running like a chicken with its head cut off."*

We agreed to Dad's terms. We set our kittens down in the grass and ran into the house to get little saucers of milk. Mother began plucking the bird. Dad walked over to the hose to wash off the axe. When we returned to the yard the kittens stood where we had left them beside the chicken's head. They were lapping up the blood.

Lessons Learned

I WAS PLACED IN A second grade class with many other learning disabled kids. That did not mean extra services and attention as it does now. It was more about grouping slow kids with other slow kids. I matriculated through an education system that was ranked 48th in the nation. On top of being in a state with little school funding, our local Washington Elementary School was very poor. I was attending the poor school, in a poor state, and was a "free breakfast and free lunch" student.

Our school building was old, but I loved the architectural details. It was originally built as a high school in 1937. Not all of the rooms were air-conditioned. Our books were often years if not decades out of date. I even remember reading a science textbook that said *someday we would fly to the Moon!* Some days the teacher would walk to the front of the classroom and pull a projection screen over the outdated world map. She would roll a squeaking metal cart to the rear of the room. We would watch in awe and amazement as her deft fingers would unreel the spool of film and place it on the carriage. She would ask one of us to turn off the lights. The teacher would turn on the film projector and each dust mote would gleam in the air. Then she would advance the film, and that wondrous noise- that pleasing repetitive fftht, fftht, fftht, would fill the room.

For the next thirty minutes we would learn about big cats on the Savannah, or the division of a cell or the mathematics behind the construction of large buildings. For thirty minutes the room would cease to be a slightly musty space filled with chalk dust, but instead became a theatre. As a child, I would smile in delight on movie days, and be so thankful that the projector worked and the film did not break. Our teachers did not have many resources and did the best they could with their meager funds and old equipment. They taught us many lessons that don't come out of books. They taught us about perseverance, ingenuity and the proper care of our bodies.

Those teachers had so little funding, but they had time. They took that time and taught us many lessons that don't fit within the current common core. They taught us about health. They taught us about food choices and exercise. They gave us dye tablets to see the plaque build-up on our teeth. They taught us how our bodies work. Indeed, my mother did not explain the process of menstruation to me. My fifth grade teacher did. She did that in a room filled with 40 girls using a film projector and a 1970's film reel. She then handed out female care packages to every girl, carefully explaining tampons versus panty liners and saying that the decision of which product to use would be up to us.

In third grade, we were taught the correct procedure for a lice check. The teacher had us disinfect our blunted pencils using alcohol. Then we would pick another child for a partner. The partner would sit in front of us faced away with their head bowed low. We would begin at the nape of the neck, lifting layer after layer of hair using our pencils like prized forensic tools. Silence would descend throughout the room as each pair searched for the tell-a-tale sign of nits or lice. It was wonderful and empowering. For the next few weeks "lice check" became the most popular playground activity, replacing string games, finger catchers and double-dutch.

Not all memories were so kind. I still remember "pee" boy from third grade. This unfortunate child had told the teacher he really needed to go the restroom. She did not let him go. He finally could not hold it anymore and urinated all over himself and his seat. For the rest of the year he lost his name; he became "pee" boy. Months after this incident, the gym coach decided to start teaching all of us ballroom dance. The room quickly paired off, leaving "pee" boy sitting on the floor, his face flushed with embarrassment. I was poor and pudgy and had all the grace of an elephant, but I walked over to him and held his hand. I thought the worse thing they can do is call me "pee boy's girlfriend." We danced.

In third grade, I was cast as the lead in our elementary school musical. I was the witch in "The Witches Brew." This was a big part with lots of singing. I was so excited I got the part, especially since ... I couldn't sing. What I mean to say is, I could belt out the songs; but had absolutely no sense of pitch or tune. So imagine my joy and surprise at being cast! I loved to sing; I just wasn't any good at it.

A few weeks into rehearsal, I accidently overheard my music teacher talking to another instructor. She told the other teacher, "Yeah, Regina's singing is horrible! I cast her because she is LOUD. It is more important to be heard, then to be able to sing at the elementary school level." I quietly slipped out. It was very hard to go to sleep that night. I wondered if I could go on stage, in front of all those people, knowing I was terrible. I decided to concentrate on the good part. I was loud. I would be very good at being loud.

This is an important lesson to learn in life. We cannot change a lot of what happens to us, but we can choose to always look on the bright side. Even when you are hit by tragedy, you can decide to take on the world and make it a better place. I may not be a good singer. But I am loud. Sometimes it is more important to be loud. It helps to get the message across. God doesn't care if the trumpet is shining and bright. He doesn't even care if it is in tune. He just needs it to be loud.

The day of the play my mother took off work to help me get into costume. She struggled to help me with my witch make-up. She tried to help me into my dime store plastic costume. When she was supposed to attach my long witch fingernails, I could see she was very frustrated. She was not sure of how to proceed. Her eyes held a film of tears, and I knew she wanted to cry. She quietly seethed instead. She was older and poorer than the other mothers who sashayed by us helping their children into fancy costumes. They did not offer to help. Mom finally finished helping me into costume and before leaving to join the audience said quietly, "I will never do this again." She never did. She never came to help with school parties or help backstage in the many plays in my future. She was made to feel unwanted and small. She would never return.

I learned a lot of lessons while in my youth. Some came from books and some came from life. I learned that without insurance when you got sick, you just suffered. I vividly remember ear infections and tonsil infections that were suffered through. I remember my mother rubbing my neck and chest with Vic's Vapor Rub in an attempt to deal with my chest colds. I even remember her dosing me with "green drops," an old cure from her childhood. I mean literally from her childhood. The bottle was from the 1930's, and I was sick in 1980. As it was still liquid and still lime green, I must assume it was very high in its alcohol content. She poured it in my ears and gave me a spoonful with sugar by mouth. The bottle advertised the many ways of administering the treatment. It did me no harm, but I am not sure it helped me. Perhaps it helped my mother. She must have been so worried and knew she could not afford the doctor's bill.

Lack of insurance affects children in other ways. I remember the day I came home from school and asked to be on the soccer team. I was told no. The family could not afford the uniforms and fees let alone the injuries sports would entail. Even physical education class or recess was problematic, as eventually you would be injured. I broke two pairs of glasses, broke my fingers, and badly sprained my wrist at school, only to be berated for hours by an abusive father. "Don't you know how much this will cost us?" he screamed.

Speaking of abuse, who recognizes the signs of abuse better than a doctor or a nurse? If medical practitioners could have seen me regularly, they would have seen the welts and bruises on my legs and arms. Would they have quietly asked the right questions? Could those questions have released me from years of torment? But alas, as an uninsured child this opportunity was denied me.

Who addresses the psychological torture of lack of appropriate treatment? I used to try to sleep while worrying about broken fingers. Would they always be crooked? Would the other children make fun of me? I remember the day I badly sprained my ankle. I could barely walk. My mother wrapped my ankle in an Ace bandage. Then my grandpa loaned me his geriatric walker so I could go to school. I begged my mom for crutches instead. "I am sorry", she said, "We cannot afford it." My face burned with shame as I hobbled down the hall with a walker too big for me to use. As the snickers echoed down the hall, I wanted to die. Why did life have to be this hard?

Of all the lessons I learned as I child, I learned the most important things in church. I would sit beside my mother on the pew and draw on my children's bulletin in order to channel my excess energy in a positive direction. I know it is important to pay attention in church, but I thought God would not mind if I drew pictures from the Bible. Even though my mother often wondered why I couldn't keep still and quiet like my little sister, she treasured these church drawings. She still keeps some of them in her hope chest.

Ten years ago my elder son Freddie took up my habit of drawing in church. During one service, I looked down to see a peculiar picture on his drawing pad. The picture consisted of a series of small houses lined up along the bottom of the paper. Above the houses stood stick people and fish in the sky. Along the very top of the page was an elongated oval. I was stumped trying to figure out the meaning of this rendering. In my best church whisper I asked, "What are you drawing?" He looked at me as though I was being particularly dull and said, "Noah's ark...from below."

In my years of teaching art, I have seen many versions of Noah's ark. Each picture contained a boat, animals, and a sunny blue sky. I never saw a picture of what lies beneath until Freddie's drawing. I guess it is just a matter of perspective. Both images are equally valid and each focuses on a different part of the story. Life is a picture painted from different perspectives. Some moments are bright and beautiful. Some are so very dark. What you see depends on where you stand.

I attended Vacation Bible School throughout my childhood. We called it VBS and I think it was the first acronym I ever used. My sister Esther and I attended many Vacation Bible School sessions, each lasting a week. We went to the various programs held by The Catholic Church, the Assembly of God, the Episcopalians, the Nazarenes and the Baptists. There were many reasons to enjoy VBS. One reason was that we were hungry and the teachers fed us Kool-Aid and cookies. Another reason was we were away from Dad and his endless chores and harsh punishments. But I think our favorite reason was because Esther and I won all the prizes. Esther and I were being raised Lutheran by our mother. We were the only Lutherans in town as far as we knew. Mom drove 31 miles once a month to Okmulgee, Oklahoma, so we could attend Trinity Lutheran Church. I did not know a lot about Martin Luther as a child, but I knew this: we were supposed to read our Bible and know what the words meant. We also were supposed to memorize a lot of verses. This helped us a great deal when we attended Vacation Bible School.

My favorite VBS was at Immanuel Lutheran Church in Breckenridge, Oklahoma. Breckenridge is a very small town surrounded by miles and miles of red dirt roads and wheat farms. Most of the roads in town are gravel and the population has stayed right around 250 since 1970. I loved this little Church and I loved the kind Pastor who preached there with his gentle, soft voice. His name was Pastor Kjergaard. He wore his clothes nicely pressed and often wore a sweater over his clerical garb. His dress and manner reminded me of Mr. Rogers from PBS. Every year he would welcome all the children in the VBS who had left backyards and toys to sit upon a pew on a summer day.

Each year he would open a large picture folio and tell us the story of the hen. I would settle into my pew as Pastor recited a story he had told since the 1950's. I loved the vivid perfection of each large illustration. He told us about the farmer who took care of the farm and the kind mother hen who lived there. He showed us panels of her proudly walking with her chicks around her whilst pecking at the food.

Then he showed a picture of the hen house catching fire. Then my eyes would well with tears as I thought of the pain the hen must endure. I had played with matches, so I was well aware of how much burns hurt. All the children would sit in rapt attention as they waited for Pastor to tell us the fate of the little loyal hen.

The next day the farmer found her. Her feathers burnt, she lay slouched over on the ground. He gingerly pushed at her and was amazed to find all of her chicks still alive beneath her scorched body. She sacrificed her life to save them.

The children in my pew would sniffle and press their hands quickly against watering eyes. Then Pastor would thank us each for coming and remind us every day to "Please bring one more friend tomorrow." He would ask, "Could you each just bring one more? Bring just one more to celebrate with us." Each day they did. A child who only attended one day was as welcome as a child who attended all five. Pastor never worried about whether we would have enough food or lesson sheets to share. Money could be stretched if needed; the most important thing was to welcome everyone to the table. In town of only 260 people we would routinely have 60-70 children in by the end of the week.

Sometimes I would ask our cousins to attend with us if they were visiting from their home in Nebraska. My mother was second youngest in her family so most of my cousins were adults, but mother had a younger brother named Gerald. Gerald was the only brother who did not follow in his father's steps and become a farmer. He went to college instead and became a principal. He and his wife Judy had five children. Three of the children were older than we were and two were younger. The family was so much fun and jolly to be around. Uncle Gerald and Aunt Judy were my Godparents or Sponsors. I was very honored to have them as Godparents as they were both very dedicated to the faith. I would sometimes get jealous of my sister though. Her Sponsors were Aunt Bertha and Aunt Minnie and they gave her toys and dolls on her birthday. My Uncle Gerald and Aunt Judy gave me prayer books.

But for my eighth birthday they gave me my most prized possession. They gave me an orange t-shirt emblazoned with the name of the sports team at their school. "The Lutheran Tigers," it said. I loved that shirt and wore it as much as I could. My father hated it. He thought my uncle was over-educated and uppity. He thought the t-shirt was a dig at him and our family. Dad said he hated uptight know-it-all Lutherans.

Dad made fun of Mom and her pious ways. He placed statues of idols and symbols of other faiths on her china cabinet next to her few knick-knacks on display. He made us children sit for hours while he read from the Bible with his own skewed interpretation. He told us God sanctified him and all his actions were pure and blessed. He could do no harm. Mom knew better though. She kept her few prized possessions locked in her hope chest or buried in her closet. She knew better than to place them in the way of Dad's fiery temper.

That was the one lesson I refused to learn.

The Power Of Creation

LOOKING BACK AT MY SECOND year of first grade, I remember only one bright spot. The entire class was creating a huge diorama for Thanksgiving. It was the moment the Pilgrims and Indians celebrate the first Thanksgiving. We were supposed to help create a forest scene and a village scene. I despaired that I had nothing to add. My Dad held up a clothespin and said, "You can add this." I furrowed my brow and asked, "Why put a clothespin in a forest scene?" Dad snapped the clothespin apart and discarded the wooden sides. Then he handed me the metal spring. "Because it is not a clothespin," he said. "It is a bear trap." In that moment, my mind slipped its moorings as he taught me creativity. I never looked at the world the same way again. Creation served me well; I managed to pass first grade on my second attempt.

In the summer of 1980, I remember endless days of sorting through piles of junk in our back yard. My sister, my brother, and I would sort as the sun beat down upon us. We would even sift organic compost from our garden pile until it was soft and dark with the rotting parts removed. Then we would then fill bags of this 'black-gold' to sell in Dad's flea-market stall. This was hot exhausting work. My father was a very hard man to live with, but even he could see we would work more productively in the shade. So he built a shed. The shed was a simple affair. It had four posts at the corners and one back wall. It was made from scrap lumber with a corrugated sheet metal roof and a workbench placed against the back wall. It was far cooler to work inside the shed, but the shed was not very pretty.

Unfortunately, we lived next to a church. Parishioners were always asking us to get rid of the junk in our yard and every couple of years a committee would come over and ask to buy our house. They wanted to raze our house and expand. Every time the committee came by my grandpa would say no. Sometimes they were told no by my Grandpa while he held a shotgun across his lap. I do not think they liked that very much. In an attempt to be good neighbors, we planted creeping vines, morning glories and honey-suckle all along our five-foot high fence. Due to the relatively temperate climate of Oklahoma, the vines obscured our yard for most of the year; but they could still see our junk sometimes and they could see our shed. One day a town official came to our yard and told us there had been a complaint. He asked, "Have you built a shed without a permit?" Dad said he didn't know he needed a permit to build a shed. Well, ignorance of the law was no excuse. We had to tear down the shed.

That meddling made Dad really angry. Dad decided to make a state-ment. He took the wood and scraps from the shed, and combining it with even more junk built a modern art installation. It was a huge cart to Calvary made of trash wood and metal and topped with a large cross and he parked in our front lawn in plain view of the church. He told the town paper it was a statement about the hostage crisis in Iran and in part it was. It made the front cover of the Sapulpa Herald. The neighbors couldn't do a thing about it, as there was no zoning code that forbade junk-art installations. My father had made his point, and my siblings and I went back to sort junk in the simmering sunlight of our backyard.

Looking back at this time in my father's life I think he was having a manic phase. He was producing a great deal of art, rarely sleeping, and drinking copious amounts of alcohol. It was a very stressful time for the entire family. Dad wrote poetry daily and was trying to get the work copyrighted. Soon after creating the cart, my father decided to paint an interpretive political mural of the coming end-times all over our kitchen. This was a very cruel thing to do to my mother and grandpa. My mother had never felt at home in her father-in-law's house. She spent as much time as she could in her bedroom, but the necessity of cooking for all of us meant a great deal of her time was spent in the kitchen. Grandpa or "Krackaw," as we all called him, sat all day in the kitchen playing solitaire. It was his favorite space in our home.

The mural was *designed to disturb*. Dad painted part of the ceiling black and created a space scene. He painted and drew with black Sharpie marker all over the room. He drew women's legs in fishnet stockings, geometric patterns, disembodied eyes, and a large piece he called the history of the world. Everywhere you looked within our kitchen there were scrawled words and an insanity of shapes and color. It was a very powerful piece and would have been edgy as street art. But in the close confines of a kitchen it was somewhat terrifying.

Dad's art began to spread throughout the house. He proceeded to "improve" the landscape prints that hung in the dining room and living room. Mom liked pastoral prints or pictures of barns and Dad had brought many such pictures home from the flea market. The prints usually were harmless artistic renderings that you would find in a hotel or a restaurant, but most of the images had dense forests in the background or trees surrounding the object of interest.

In those forests Dad drew eyes. You would not notice them at first, and then you would. Then they could not be unseen. That might seem like a joke in a postmodern world where computer sites like Pinterest abound with 1970s prints that are gleefully over-painted with Eldritch Abominations, but to a little girl they were terrifying. It did not help that dad would tell us they were "Treetop Boogers." Dad would tell us backwoods tales from his youth about Jibone, Boogerjack and the Treetop Boogers. Jibone and Boogerjack were just bootleggers who got into all kinds of trouble, but the Treetop Boogers were monsters that lived in the tree branches. You could only see their eyes. Once, Mom left home early in the morning to attend a funeral. She did not tell us why she was leaving before she left and would not return till well after dark. Dad had us convinced that the Treetop Boogers had gotten her. We cried with joy that night when she finally came in the door, as we were very worried that we had lost her.

In addition to Dad writing poetry, he liked to read poetry to us all. Dad began reading us *Beowulf* with its gory woodcut imagery of monster and man. He read it several times and I was somewhat fixated by the power of the poem's narrative combined with such gruesome art. When my teacher asked our elementary school class to name books that each student found especially interesting, I responded, "*Beowulf.*" My teacher knew I was a very poor reader and she quizzed me about the plot in disbelief. I told her about the hero defeating Grendel, then fighting Grendel's monstrous mother, and finally succumbing to the wounds from the dragon. The other children just looked at me quizzically and listed much more traditional titles.

Dad's creative phase turned dark as winter approached. He drank even more and would insult my mother and my grandfather on a daily basis. I would avoid him when I could and tolerate his tirades when unable to escape his presence. One evening he began to fixate on destroying my favorite t-shirt that depicted the Lutheran Tigers soccer team. He teased me and goaded me about it. He told me I looked fat in it and said I could never succeed at sports and should not wear it. He demanded I find it and give it to him. I searched throughout my room and could not find it. My mother took me aside and whispered it was safe in the dryer. I looked at her with such intensity knowing nothing was ever safe in this house. I whipped around. I raced over to the dryer and dug it out. I thrust it in my father's face. "Here it is!" I yelled. "Here is my shirt!"

He smiled a crooked smile and pulled out his pocketknife. He shredded my favorite possession right before my eyes. In that moment, my mind crystalized with a white-hot anger as he taught me the power of destruction. I never looked at the world the same way again. The lesson of destruction served me well. I learned that there are people in this world who exist in order to break you down. I will not let them win.

The Impala

By 1980 the '76 Impala had a lot of miles on it. Its exterior suffered wear and the paint was beginning to peel. The inside was immaculate though. When Mom and Dad purchased the car they had the seats wrapped in plastic. It made for scorching hot seats in the summer and freezing cold seats in the winter, but the interior upholstery was spotless. That was pretty amazing, as both my brother and sister were prone to carsickness. The car held up very well to their frequent bouts of vomiting on Dad's spontaneous road trips.

Dad would often get an itch to travel, so he would pack all of us into the car and just drive. Sometimes it went well and we would end up at a museum or park. Sometimes the family would just ride in the car for hours trapped upon those plastic seats. We would listen to Dad preach his version of reality and harangue us for our many faults. I would look out the window and try not to listen. Dad would rant about the Jews, the blacks, the world that kept him down, the stupidity of his wife and children, and our holier-than-thou relatives. Mom would softly say, "Now, Gilmer..." in a defeated voice. But Dad would never stop his tirades.

I hated those rides with the family, but the rides alone with Dad were so much worse. The rides began in the second year of first grade. At first I suppose I felt a bit special being asked to go alone to the store or the Prattville Flea market. Even when your Dad is a monster you wanted to love him and hoped to be loved in return. Soon he was telling me I was pretty and perhaps I would like to have a new doll. I loved dolls. Soon he began to ask me what I knew about the birds and the bees. I started to feel very small in the large backseat of the Impala. I sat as far away from him as I could. I sat in the plastic covered backseat on the right and pressed my body close to the door.

He angled the rearview mirror so he could see me and I could see his eyes. Then he began to make his case about my duty as his daughter. He told me what the other girls did for their fathers. They would take their pants down and sit upon their father's laps. He told me just the other day he walked in on my seven-year-old neighbor loving her Daddy. She was sitting on her Daddy with no clothes on. She must really love her Daddy. He asked if I would do that for him. I said quietly, "No." I looked out the window. I looked at the knob that you would press to lock the door. It looked like a font in miniature. It stood tall, silver and pure upon the door. I imagined it filled with holy water. I imagined a little me praying there.

He told me Mommy was getting older and rarely loved him. I could love him he said. He looked at me in the rear view mirror. "You know your Mom works hard and is tired. You could make her life easier. It will be our little secret. You just have to say yes." I told Dad no. I told Dad no so many times. I tried to never be left alone with him. Whenever I failed, he would try to touch me or show me pages of pornography and suggest I do the things pictured.

This went on for months. Then one day it was so very cold. Dad said he was taking me to the flea market to work. So I went in my room and put on my thermal underwear underneath my jeans so I would not freeze in the market stall. But he did not take me to the flea market. He took me to a store where there were row upon row of dolls. He told me, "Pick whichever doll you like. But after we buy it, you have to do whatever I ask." As we walked toward the counter, I filled with fear. The lines were so long it must have been close to Christmas. Dad got angry and impatient. He threw my doll to the ground and we left the store. I walked beside him numbly and sat inside the Impala. He drove us to Lake Sahoma and parked among the barren trees. I looked out the window at a forest of switches poking out of the dirty snow. He told me to take off my pants. I said, "No, I have thermal underwear on." He said take those off too. He said I didn't need to take off my coat to have sex, just my pants.

I felt the blood bang upon my eardrums and my body tense with anger and fear. Then I began to scream, "I hate you! I hate you! We all hate you! Everyone hates you!" He turned and glared at me. He said with gritted teeth, "I am going to cut a switch and then I am going to come back to the car. If you do not take those pants down then, I will beat you bloody." Dad got out the door and slammed it. Then I began to pray. I prayed like I had never prayed before. I thought of that story in the Bible, the story of Abraham and Isaac. I thought how the preachers told it wrong. They always said that Abraham was delivered of his horrible task, but I knew the one who truly prayed upon that alter was Isaac.

I looked into the wood where Dad was madly hacking at tree covered in ice. I shook back and forth in my seat my body propelled in constant litany of bargains with God. "Please God, Please God help me. Help me. Help me. I promise I will be good. I will make it up to you. Just help me now...." I looked out of my window rapidly clouding from the condensation of my whispered prayers. I watched my father attack a branch in anger. Then the knife slipped and Dad had a large gash on his hand. He quickly wrapped his handkerchief around the wound and walked to the car. He said a few choice curses and we drove home. On the ride home, I silently thanked God for deliverance, for sparing me as he had spared Isaac. When we arrived I shook as I walked in the house.

Inside the radio was on and it was warm. Esther was reading a book and Eugene was watching TV. Krackcaw was playing solitaire at the kitchen table. The house did nothing to acknowledge my horror and fright.

I walked with Dad to the bathroom. I helped Dad dress his wound. As I put the last Band-Aid on he looked at me. His face was sad and his eyes looked broken "Do you really hate me? " he asked. I looked into the pale blue eyes of this very troubled man and said, "No, Daddy, I love you." Then I put the Band-Aid box back in the cabinet and walked away.

That was that. We never spoke of that day in the car again.

I would not let myself be alone with him after that day. From that moment on I watched him and tried to protect my sister and my friends. I did my best to make sure they did not suffer as I did. But I was only a child and I did not succeed in protecting everyone from Dad. During winter break I told my Aunt Minnie that Dad was after me, and I was sure he would try for Esther next. She listened and decided to tell my Mother.

I remember watching from my Aunt Minnie's glass front door as Mom packed the Impala for our return trip to Sapulpa. Aunt Minnie had a transparent decal of a Monarch butterfly on her glass door. I would watch Mom through the rippling orange of a butterfly's wing. I could not hear what words were said, but I watched my Mother's face screw up as she began to cry. I watched my Aunt Minnie hold her as she sobbed. Aunt Minnie and Aunt Hilda came up with a plan. Esther and I would spend summers with them. If we were never left alone with Dad he would not be able to hurt us. From the age of nine to the age of fifteen, my sister and I would spend every summer with our Aunts.

I would thank God for this solution, but miracles come at a price. Three weeks into our first summer with our Aunts, we were able to call our Mom. Long distance calls were expensive and infrequent in those days. We had never been away from our mother before. We excitedly told her about all we had done in Enid. We told her we loved her and that we were being good.

Then we asked about our pet cats.

Months and months had passed since the day we had found them in the trash. Esther named her cat Snow White and she was a lovely white and gray feline. I had named my striped kitten Sleeping Beauty as I did not know he was a tom. When he reached maturity he ran away. So Esther and I shared Snow White. Snow White never went to a vet so she was never fixed. It was not long before she had kittens. Esther and I did our best to give the kittens away, but when we left for the summer there were still two kittens left at home. We asked our mother how Snow White and the kittens were doing?

There was a pause on the line. Mother softly said we were not there to feed them or take care of them. She told us Dad had killed them by chopping off their heads and buried their bodies in the backyard. Snow White yowled in sorrow and would not stop. She was shot and buried beside the kittens.

I cried so hard that night. I had failed in my responsibility. No matter how hard I tried I could not protect everyone from Dad.

The Twins

OUR WORLD WAS A SMALL one when I was a child in Sapulpa. If I went out of my door and veered right, within a few blocks I would end up at Davis Park. There I would play in the small creek or upon the metal play structures that gleamed in the summer sun. If I went out my front door and walked to my left, I would quickly end up in our small downtown business district. If I could fly like bird far above my small figure walking upon the buckled pavement of my youth, I would see the spires of all the churches that surround us. I would see my little green home with its junk-filled yard and its enormous pecan tree whose canopy stretched over most of the lot. A block away there was another house painted white with cool blue gray paint on the floor of the front porch. It was a majestic house. A cat named Tiger lived there. In this house the light streamed in through the living room sheers. The staircase was regal, but that did not stop little girls from riding mattresses down its bumpy length.

My best friends, the twins, lived within this house.

I met one of the twins on my way home from school when I was only six years old. She stood beneath a stop sign and smiled. She was one of two, but I did not know that then. We talked shyly as strange children are wont to do. She said she lived in the big white house on the hill with her twin sister and the rest of her family. Angie and Katie Berg became fast friends with my sister Esther and me. We spent many years walking to Washington Elementary School together. We were all in the same grade, and they were as much a pair as my sister and I.

The twins lived a hard life. They were the last children of a dying marriage. They lived in the big house with five siblings and their mother. We rarely saw their Mom as she mostly stayed in her room. She was stuck fast inside by grief of life lived not as intended. We worried about the twins. My sister Esther and I were poor, but there was always food in our fridge, not so Katie and Angie. Many times I opened their fridge to find pickle juice, condiments, and nothing else. Or I would watch them live for days on only fried bologna. My mother would press food into their hands every time she saw them, saying softly, "Those poor girls."

Angie and Katie continued to play with us as the years passed. Even with all their struggles, the twins did well in school. They played sports and had lots of friends. They even had a paper route that occasionally Esther and I would help them with. We so enjoyed rolling up the papers and binding them with rubber bands. The ink from the typeface turned our hands as black as the asphalt turned the soles of our feet. We split the heavy canvas messenger bags among the four of us and would run for blocks throwing the papers toward doors and over fences. The twins appreciated our help on these delivery days, but they needed us when it was time to collect the monthly subscription fee.

It was dangerous collecting newspaper subscriptions funds. Some families had mean guard dogs and some folks did not want to pay, but that is not the reason we needed four of us to collect the monies. We had to watch out. If all of us stood upon the stoop, we were not easy targets. We waited patiently together, knowing there was safety in numbers and always refusing offers to come inside. We were very aware of stranger danger and had at times avoided being grabbed by only quick reflexes and solidarity.

Subscription collection happened only once a month, but the twins played with us daily. Children don't do so well at constant vigilance. We most often would play at the twins' house, but sometimes they came to our backyard. We would play town, circus and build castles in our sand-box. We would play and Dad would watch us.

Media Matters

By the summer of 1982, Esther and I were used to spending June through August with our Aunts in Enid, Oklahoma. We missed the twins and worried, but tried to make new friends on the quiet cul-de-sac. We kept very busy. We would spend days with Aunt Minnie and nights with Aunt Hilda across the street. They would teach us so many things. They would send us to camp Lutherhoma and buy our fall school clothes each year. Aunt Minnie was so happy to care for us. My sister Esther was her Goddaughter and was like the child she never had. Esther was always small for her age so she would cuddle in Aunt Minnie's lap.

Each Tuesday night we volunteered with Aunt Hilda at "Project Philip." There we mailed Bible study packets to men in prison. Esther and I would stand in the back of the room and sing hymns as we stuffed hundreds of mailers. We helped with many church events and often we went to the movies. In the years prior to 1982, we had seen only one movie in the theatre and that film was *Darby O'Gill and the Little People*. It was a rather terrifying choice for a Saturday matinee film. Once the banshee appeared, my sister dove under her theatre seat and would not come out for the rest of the movie.

1982 was replete with amazing cinematic choices. Our Aunt Minnie and Aunt Hilda took us to *E.T. The Extraterrestrial*. That was very kind because they really did not enjoy science fiction. They also took us to see *Annie* which all of us enjoyed immensely! When Esther and I began dressing up like Miss Hannigan and the orphans, my Aunt Hilda bought us a vinyl record of the soundtrack so we could sing all the songs again and again and again. My Aunts were very patient and loving women. Our Aunts also had cable television, so when we were not belting out show tunes we were immersing ourselves in a fairly constant stream of 1970's television. I have heard television described as an opiate of the masses or as a method of escapism. It can be that and as Jerry Seinfeld would say, "Not that there is anything wrong with that." Sometimes we need to escape even if it is only during one hour of prime time.

At home in Sapulpa, my sister Esther and I had an old black & white TV set in our bedroom. We would turn the channel with pliers as the turning knob had fallen off years before. An old metal clothes hanger was jammed in the back of the set in an often-vain attempt to pick up the UHF channels. We counted ourselves lucky to have this small static-filled escape within our room. Periodically, I see articles in the press condemning screen use in a child's bedroom. I'll bet that those who condemn never used a television to drown out the horror that awaited right outside that bedroom. But television offered so much more than escapist fare; the medium taught us. People have often asked me, "Who taught you how to be an empowered patient?" I respond the television of the 1970s and 80s did.

To me Grandma Walton from *The Waltons* (1971-1981) is the face of a stroke. I was only six years old when Grandma Walton came back on the show after Ellen Corby, the actress playing the role, suffered a stroke in 1977. I remember the shock of seeing her face and words twisted, but I also remember my joy upon seeing her return. This was 1978, years before ADA (Americans with Disabilities Act) legislation; it was not common to see people with disability or illness on TV. I was only six, but I was proud of Grandma Walton. I was proud of what she stood for. I took her bravery very personally. My mother had an episode of Bell's palsy during that year. My mother no longer smiled. Half of her face was slack and she wore bandage over one eye to keep it moist. Small children would point at her in the grocery store, but each day my mother would go out and live her life bravely just like Grandma Walton.

I also watched episode after episode of *Quincy, ME,* (1976-1983). Yes, I was a nine-year-old who enjoyed forensic science. I was very impressed by Quincy, long before I learned that the actor who played a doctor on television had testified before Congress. Jack Klugman and his show, with its depiction of patients who have rare diseases, helped to pass the Orphan Drug Act in 1983. This piece of legislation would guarantee access to needed drugs for thousands of Americans in the years to come.

I did not know it then, but I was also watching my future husband's favorite show on a regular basis. *M.A.S.H.* (1972-1983) was a funny sardonic show and many of the jokes went far over my head, but I did enjoy it. I was very impressed by that show's brave decision to dedicate the majority of its final episode, *"Goodbye, Farewell and Amen,"* to Dr. Hawkeye Pierce's nervous breakdown and hospitalization for mental treatment. This helped promote a greater awareness of the effects of mental illness and depression and showcased a potential road to recovery. This episode aired in 1983 and was the most watched television broadcast in the history of American television until 2010. I was 10 years old at the time that it aired, but I vividly remember sometimes a "chicken" is not a chicken. In that episode, Hawkeye is on a bus surrounded by civilians as the enemy is patrolling close by. One woman holds a chicken on her lap and it won't stop clucking. Hawkeye commands her to make the chicken be silent. She suffocates the chicken in her arms. As the episode progresses, the audience realizes it was not a chicken. She had suffocated her own baby. The doctor had caused harm and he had to deal with that. Sometimes the choices we make in life can lead to someone else's death.

My favorite program was *The Incredible Hulk* (1978-1982). I have always loved superheroes, especially ones that are portrayed with such depth of character. I also cherished that no matter how mad the hulk was he would never hurt an innocent. In addition to the action scenes expected in such a program, this series depicted the sorrow and grief upon losing a spouse. I started watching The Incredible Hulk at the age of five and I could not wait for each episode to begin. The program conquered topic after harsh topic. I was only 7 years old when the episode "Metamorphosis" aired. In less than one hour, the show addressed anger issues, classism, drug abuse and passive suicide. It promoted altruism and the concept of embracing your calling in life, regardless of whether or not it is economically advantageous.

The television program that affected me the most in a medical way was *Little House on the Prairie* (1974-1983). When I was young, I needed glasses. But I didn't know I needed glasses. I had gotten used to not being able to see very well. I spent second and third grade squinting at the chalkboard during class. I would try to sit close so I could see what was written on the wall. One afternoon as Esther and I watched television, an episode of Little House on the Prairie aired. In this episode, the character Mary was squinting and pulling at her eyes. She needed glasses. I told my Mom, "I need glasses just like Mary." She said, surely not, as I was only in fourth grade at the time. I told her I was doing everything Mary was doing within the episode. A couple of weeks later my Mother got me an appointment to see an eye doctor.

I had been to a doctor before. When I was sick the doctor spent most of his talking with my mother. He would give me a quick look over and tell mother what he was prescribing to make me better. The eye doctor was very different. He had me sit straight up in a chair that looked like a throne. I would rest my chin in a special cup. Then he slid circular panes of glass before my eyes. Then he began the calming repetitive litany familiar to all of those who suffer from bad eyesight.

"Is this better, or this one? One or two, A or B?" Again and again the glass panes slid in place and the litany continued. Again and again I was forced to choose between this form of blurry and that form of blurry. I was amazed at a dawning realization that came over me. Through it all, I was in charge. These glass plates would change, would flip, would slide into place because of the nimble fingers of a doctor who listened patiently to a ten-year-old. After countless queries of "this... now this," the glass panes slid into place with a metallic click and I could see. One week later my glasses arrived. I went outside and I saw the trees. The trees had leaves again. For many years, distant trees had only been crowned with a glory of impressionistic green. Now the leaves were back, because I had new eyes.

With my new glasses firmly in place, my sister Esther and I watched a lot of programs designed for children. Even though I was ten, I loved Mr. Rodgers, his train, and his kind puppets. I always felt very safe watching the show. My favorite children's program was *Sesame Street* (1969-) When I heard the song begin "Sunny Days sweeping the clouds away..." I would run in and sit on the floor in front of the TV mesmerized by Big Bird, Oscar the Grouch and Snuffleupagus. I grew up watching Sesame Street and fell in love with the idea of living in a city. As an adult, I would decide to live in a bustling city for 16 years. I watched felted monsters and people peacefully coexist, and as an adult I paint diversity. I watched adults refuse to see "Snuffleupagus," so I now mention the elephant in the room every chance I get. Today if you watch Sesame Street the adults do see Snuffleupagus. After 17 seasons the writers decided the gag must go. It was more important for children to know that the adults would believe them if they were speaking the truth, even if that truth was a hard thing say. Even if that truth was about the abuse the child was suffering.

Sharks In Jars

IN THE FALL OF 1982, we returned home with new school clothes, rested bodies and cherished souls. Life was still hard but we were buoyed by the refreshing summer behind us. I felt very sorry for my fifteen-year-old brother Eugene. He stayed at home while Esther and I spent the summers in Enid, but it was the best solution we had at the time.

This is the fall I entered fourth grade. This was a very big step in our school. Fourth and fifth graders attended class on the second floor in the highest classrooms. I felt happy to be up so high and look out windows to see blue sky. The second year of first grade in the dank basement seemed so long ago. This was a very special year. I went from being child who struggled with reading, spelling and math, to being an above average student. This dramatic change was due, in large part, to Mrs. Graham, my fourth grade teacher. Mrs. Graham was a thoughtful teacher with the personal resources to bedeck her room with astounding things. Her classroom was filled with plants and books and sharks in jars.

Yes, sharks in jars. A large shelf along the wall had deli-size pickle jars filled with formaldehyde. Within these jars sharks and deep-sea specimens would float. The light pouring through the classroom window would shine through the cloudy ethereal liquid.   There was another world inside those jars, a world far away from alcoholic fathers and walls that weep. This was a world of crystal blue oceans and summer deep-sea dives. I would stare at the jars for hours and would see beyond the floating deathly stillness. I would not sorrow for the baby shark, its life cut short; I would marvel that there was another day and another way to live.

In this reverie, Mrs. Graham spoke to me. She understood that I was not dumb, merely struggling. She created an IEP (Individual Education Plan) for me years before I would understand what those initials meant. She went back to the beginning, to *cat* and *sat*, while my peers worked on words like *encyclopedia*. She would draw happy faces on my homework and tests, as I turned in the work of a first grader in a room of fourth graders.

She taught me how to shine.

It felt odd to be good at school. I had been a failure for so long. I had failed first grade and ever since had been in the same grade as my little sister. My sister Esther was very good at school. Her work was neat. She had many friends and knew *"her inside voice from her outside voice."* She was small, somewhat shy and she was an excellent student. I had been her older sister, her sometimes protector, but I had never been the smart one.

In 1983, most people did not talk about dyslexia and I could not explain why reading and writing were so hard for me. I remember telling Mrs. Graham how to spell my name on my report card and getting it wrong. I said it was *MCcanless* when it should have been McCanless. Mrs. Graham looked at me and smiled a gentle smile that caused a cascading ripple in the wrinkles on her face and she asked, "Are you sure you want it spelled that way?" When I nodded my assent, she wrote it just that way.

The next morning Esther and I hurriedly gathered our school supplies and I gave my father the report card as he sat at his writing desk. It was late fall and he had been drinking heavily. My father was furious at

the error in capitalization as he signed the card. He began to write hurt-
ful things to Mrs. Graham in the comment box. He called her names
as he wrote, cussing her out and slurring his words together. I stood
frozen. It was not her fault. I could not let my kind and loving teacher
take the blame. As my face grew red, I stammered "No, Daddy. It was
my mistake. I told her to write it that way. "

My father looked up at me. His jaw was clenched and his blue eyes
were ice. I had been brushing my hair moments before. My pink poly-
resin hairbrush lay on the table beside me. It was a pretty brush. It
was pink and translucent. The bristles were white and were sunk deep
within the resin base. Like all brushes of its ilk, it was very heavy.

Dad's hand darted like the strike of a snake. He grabbed the brush off
the table spilling my pile of schoolbooks and stuck me across the side of my
face. I fell back and out of the corner of my eye I saw my little sister Esther
escape out the front door. She ran ahead to school. Dad stood up and tow-
ered over me. He leaned in, his voice a growl as he told me my teacher was
stupid for listening to a girl who could not even spell her own name.

I crawled around the floor picking up my books and papers as I
listened to his tirade. I pulled my body away from his feet and hands. I
numbly gathered the rumpled report card and left for school. I was going be late. My shaking fingers touched the side of my face and felt the
inflamed wheal of flesh rising on my cheek.

When I got to school, I was tardy. I slowly climbed those stairs that I
so proudly mounted at the start of my fourth grade year. When I reached
the top stop step, I stood within a shaft of morning light. I watched the
particles of dust ebb and flow. I sat down on that stop step and softly
cried. My fingers began to trace the indented lines of the rubber stair-
well tread. Thus seated, I waited in the hall for Mrs. Graham. When
a fellow student alerted her to my presence, I apologized for the sad

condition of my report card and for my father's comments. I explained that I had gotten in trouble for my incorrect capitalization, hence my swollen face. Mrs. Graham sat beside me on the top stair step. She held my hand and said she would help me.

I sat beside her for an eternity as the dust motes rose and fell within the beams of light. My fingers traced a meditation on that stairway tread as my fellow students sat within the classroom, copying line after line of spelling words. Time seemed to stop within our makeshift hall-way confessional as I told Mrs. Graham about fists and switches. I spoke of fathers who tell their daughters the stories of the "birds and bees" when they are much too young. I used that euphemism, because even in this quiet moment of trust, admitting to being the victim of attempted incest is such a scary and taboo thing to do. I told her all these things and trusted she would find a way to help me out of this hellish life. I had never told an adult outside of my family about all the abuse I had suf-fered in my ten years. Mrs. Graham hugged me. She gave me a Kleenex to dry my tears and I went into the class.

That was that. We never spoke of that day on the stairs again.

Perhaps Mrs. Graham thought it was not her place to intercede. Perhaps she was scared of my father too. This was the time before teach-ers and doctors were required to report abuse. She really did not have to act. A little part of me began to hate Mrs. Graham. I would look at the sharks in jars and no longer think of oceans far away. I would think of being trapped. Mrs. Graham was such a nice person, but I realized be-ing nice does not always equate with acting bravely. As the years passed by my hate diminished, I looked back upon my life and realized she did try to help in her own subtle way.

In the weeks after I spoke with Mrs. Graham, a police officer visited the class. I did not realize that he probably came at Mrs. Graham's request. We often would have professionals visit in those days. The dentist came and gave us those tablets that turned our teeth pink. The fireman taught us stop, drop, and roll. The policeman spoke about abuse. He said, "Some of you may see abuse in your life. If the abuse ever becomes *too* bad, call these numbers on this card." He then proceeded to hand out a little folded card with hotline numbers for Creek County, Oklahoma.

In my years of promoting patient advocacy, I have attended many meetings focused on public health where we will begin a heated debate about the words we use in health messaging. Someone, often the facilitator, will usually try to stop further "off topic" discussion by the throwaway comment: "That is just semantics." Semantics is everything and words are powerful indeed. I sat upon a stair. I bared my soul. I recited a litany of abuse. Now I was being told that at some point in the future the abuse would become *too bad* and I could call that number. I grasped that card with such sorrow and trepidation. Why wasn't what I already suffered enough abuse? When I got home I put that card in a special place so I could use it on the auspicious day that our family's abuse became horrific.

It would be seven more years before I would call the numbers on that card.

As my fourth grade year progressed, I continued to do well in school. I brought my report cards home to my mother to sign. There were no more tear-filled confessions. A part of me still loved Mrs. Graham, but I did not trust her anymore. I had learned a final lesson from Mrs. Graham. Sometimes when your life is hellish, you have to save yourself.

Easter Mourning

I HAVE HAD MANY EASTER mornings in my life. Two have been tragic.

When my husband Fred was hospitalized in 2009, it was hard to plan for Easter. On Saturday after staying all day by Fred's side, my mother-in-law, Joan, and I stopped at a restaurant to get some dinner. While waiting for our order, I ran into a dress shop to get a new Easter dress. I wanted to look nice for Fred. I found a dress in about five minutes. It was the prettiest blue. I thought Fred would like it.   I had already purchased our sons' clothes a few weeks before, when Fred was merely "in pain" and not diagnosed with kidney cancer.

Earlier that very day, I placed 48 Easter Eggs in every corner and challenging hiding place within Fred's hospital room. I was determined we would enjoy Easter Sunday as a family no matter what.   Easter day was very hard for us. Everyone is so happy on Easter. One of my friends at church took a picture of the boys and me after the Easter service. When Fred saw the photo he told me to destroy the picture. I looked horrific. My face seemed cracked as if my life had broken in some way. My memories returning to a past I thought I had escaped.

In the spring of 1983, we celebrated Easter in our own backyard.

My sister, my brother, and I worked all day Saturday. We would spend the preceding week sorting, cleaning and packing merchandise. On Friday night we would load the truck and leave on Saturday before daybreak. Once we hit the concrete pad of our stall, Esther and I would begin setting up card table after card table. All of us would then haul heavy boxes out of the truck, being careful to hold the boxes away from our bodies as they probably contained "fiddle-back spiders." Eugene would often leave after set-up, as he was not as good at the customer service aspect of the flea market.

At the flea market we would see all sorts of folks. It is like a dark carnival. We put on the show, sell the product to the customers and do not bat an eye at the deformed of mind or body. Each weekend we would serve customers that rarely frequented traditional shops and establishments. All were welcome to roll a wheelchair onto our concrete slab and there were no doorways to impede their course. I would talk about Frankhoma pottery with a woman covered in severe burns or haggle about the price of shovels with the man whose face was a ruin of boils and warts. These daily scenes informed my childhood and taught me about the vast array of individuals who live within our world. I felt honored to help those who had suffered. Nevertheless, Esther and I were very pleased at sunset when Dad told us he would stay the night on Saturday and set up again Sunday by himself. We were able to go home a bit early.

We were excited because Sunday was Easter. I had planned an Easter egg hunt for my siblings. I boiled a bunch of eggs, painted them and hid them throughout the backyard. My mother had to work that day at the hospital. As a housekeeper, she worked most weekends. We would not be able to go to Church that day, but I thought we could still celebrate with an Easter Egg Hunt. I dressed in a very nice sundress. I asked Esther and Eugene to come out into the yard. We ran around the yard finding eggs. It was a warm and lovely day. The fence was bedecked with climbing vines and the Easter lilies had bloomed. It was hard to find the eggs amongst the vibrant colors of spring.

Then the phone rang.

My Grandpa was in the house, but he was hard of hearing so he asked me to come get the phone. Virginia Beaverson was on the line. She ran the local flea market were we worked. She said, "Regina, I have some bad news. Is your mom there?" I told Virginia that mom was at work. Virginia went on, "Well, honey your Daddy was in a knife fight with another man last night. He killed the other man and your dad was hurt real bad. They have life-flighted him to St. John's. I will try to tell your Mom at work." I numbly hung up the phone. Esther and Eugene were still playing in the yard.

When Mom had arrived at work that Sunday, she was told there was a blood trail she needed to clean up near the employee entrance. She grabbed her mop and trudged down the hall the clean up the drying blood. She did not know it was her husband's. When Dad had arrived at the hospital during the night he was very disoriented due to blood loss. Both the men in the fight had wielded knives. Dad's arm was cut severing the tendons to two fingers. He also was very nearly gutted. The other man was dead. I do not know if he died from the knifing or from Dad repeatedly running over him as he backed out of the parking lot. Dad had trouble driving due to blood loss and the need to hold his guts in with his injured hand. Mom soon found out what had happened in the night and she came home briefly. She was very scared of driving in a city, so Krackcaw drove them both. My grandpa did not always notice stop signs or stop lights so I am sure the drive was very scary. We children waited alone at home.

The following week was a trying time. The entire family waited to hear if Dad would pull through his surgeries. The stress of not knowing was hard to bear. School was also very stressful because Dad's altercation was front-page news. I remember walking to school early that week and as we approached the entrance of the building everyone stopped and stared at us. My sister Esther's teacher went to her and said that she was praying for our father. Esther told me later that she was praying too, but she was not sure that it was for healing.

Dad survived his surgeries and was placed in jail. This was a time of great peace in our home. Life was no longer lived on eggshells. We laughed and played with a semblance of stability. There was no screaming and yelling within our home. Soon Dad would go to trial. I remember wishing they would put us on the stand so I could recommend incarceration. They did not ask us to testify. Dad had a pretty good lawyer and he was convicted of Manslaughter in the second degree. He was a felon and could no longer vote or own a gun. He would be on parole for three years with time served while awaiting trial.

I was home sick from school the day Dad came home. He looked very scary as he came through the door leaning on my mother. He had a scraggly gray beard and his dental bridge was missing. His arm was pulled up against his body and his fingers on that hand were gnarled and unresponsive as they would be for the rest of his life. He saw me and began to scream obscenities at me for being home. I tried to explain I was sick. He responded I had no idea what sick was, but would find out if I did not get the hell out of that room. I hid in my room for the rest of the day. I spent the rest of my years in school trying to avoid ever taking a sick day.

The Power Of Story

IN THE SUMMER OF 1984, I would discover that television escapism has nothing on books. Now that I could read chapter books, I began to devour everything in sight. I well remember the night I found my favorite fairytale. I was to sleep in the spare bedroom in My Aunt Hilda's house. I found my Aunt's collection of Junior Classic Fairytales published in the 1950's beside her sewing box. Between the green linen covers of one book I found a Grimm's Fairytale. Mother Hulda.

I loved Mother Hulda. I loved her even though I did not know her other names: Holle, Hel, Hilda, Holda, the Goddess in three parts (Maiden, Mother, Crone), the Guardian of the Netherworld, the protector of children, the Goddess of the storm, the leader of the Wild Hunt. Mother Hulda waits at the bottom of the wishing well. She is the Goddess of spinning.

It was a tale of a young girl who must spin all day for her lazy stepsister and stepmother. She spins so much that she cuts her fingers on the spindle and covers it with blood. Her stepmother commands her to wash the spindle in the well. She tries to wash the spindle in the cool deep waters. Accidentally, she dropped it into the depths. She was filled with worry, but told her stepmother the fate of the spindle. Her stepmother tells her to jump in after it. Filled with despair she jumps into the well. Instead of splashing into the dark depths, she falls into another world. It is a beautiful world with blue skies, green grass, and flowers. She walks a while and comes upon an oven full of bread. The loaves call out, begging to be removed before they burn. The girl removes the loaves. She walks further and comes upon an apple tree. The apples beg her pick them as they are ripe. The girl picks the apples. The girl walks even further and finds a cottage with an old woman inside named Mother Hulda. She serves the old woman for weeks and weeks. Mother Hulda rewards her for her labors by showering her with gold. The girl returns to our world, and her stepsister is jealous so she jumps into the well. She doesn't save the bread and she doesn't pick the apples. She does a poor job of helping Mother Hulda. In the end, Mother Hulda covers her in tar. I loved to read this story in my bedroom at Aunt Hilda's. It was unlike any other story I had ever read. There was no prince to rescue the maiden in distress. In this story, the young girl saves herself through hard work and kindness.

As we grew older, Aunt Hilda would let us stay at Aunt Minnie's for the night. I would stay up reading much past my bedtime, sometimes hearing the garage door open at 1:00 or 2:00 am. Aunt Minnie would gently berate me and then tell me a "do not ever" story. As a nurse she saw so many things and sometimes she would come home, shake her head and say, "Do not ever jump out of a car as it is driving down the highway." Or it would be "Do not ever stick your tongue all the way into a soda can."

That fall in fifth grade our class was donated a large amount of books. I was very excited about that! We had so many books our teacher even gave us books that were in disrepair. I was given several books in our teacher's literature purge. My favorite books were all of the Little House books, A Little Princess, Pollyanna, and Heidi. These pint-sized heroines inspired me with their ability to overcome adversity. I loved the idea of imagining and then creating a beautiful world within a cold dark attic. I could envision a rainbow of color hidden in chandelier glass and play the game of always thinking of something to be glad about. I could understand the allure of returning to healthy mountain air over the coal dust vapors of a Victorian city.

We students were very pleased to have the new books, but even after purging the damaged ones we did not have enough bookshelves to shelf the remaining titles. My teacher was very enterprising though; she contacted the local lumberyard and requested they donate some two by fours and cinderblocks so we could make shelves. The lumberyard manger said yes with one caveat; we would have to pick up the supplies. I bet the manager thought the teacher would come by with a truck and pick them up.

That year our fifth grade class had a field trip.

We left the school as a class with our strong backs and eager minds. We walked to the lumberyard. Some of us grabbed the two by fours, some of us cinderblocks and some us combined the two to make a carry yoke for two students to heft. We walked those blocks all the way back to school and up three flights of stairs. Then we assembled those shelves and placed the books upon them. We stood back and looked proudly at our work. I cannot believe there was a class anywhere else in the entire nation who cherished their bookshelves as much as we did ours.

We loved those shelves because we overcame adversity and made that which we needed. It wasn't pretty, it wasn't perfect, but it was ours.

The Gun

In sixth grade, I had the pleasure of attending a newly constructed middle school. It was designed to create the best learning environment. Nothing would distract us from the written word; and so, they created a building without windows. Oh, there were these thin light aperture areas at the top of a wall. (We needed to get some sunlight after all.) But we had no view of the outside world. It felt like a prison. Children really like to see out. They will climb on top of tables or shelves to see the world around them. As adults, we often let the world grow narrow and only see what affects us directly.

I was working in the flea market stall that fall, when my father came over with a man in a hat. They told me to step into the woods with them away from the traffic of the booth. I was very frightened. No good can come from stepping into the woods. My father said, "This man here is looking to sell a gun, and seeing how I'm a felon, I can't buy it. But you can." I looked into my Father's eyes and saw little crinkles of anger at the edges.

I looked at the older man in the hat. He handed me the handgun. "Now, careful darlin,' it's loaded. Your daddy said you might want to try it out. You can shoot it right over there into the ground."

I remember many things within my life with great clarity. The bowl of yellow cornflakes I ate with my maternal grandfather when I was not quite two years old. I still see within my mind the lovely red yarn that was tied to a present from Aunt Mabel when I was but five. I can also close my eyes and see the graphite sheen of gunmetal as I pulled the trigger and shot the earth. The gun worked. My Father handed me the wad of bills, and I bought the gun.

The Christmas Tree

I LOOKED UPON THE CRUMPLED box with its porcupine interior of evergreen branches and smoothed out the bill in my hand. Scrawled in red sharpie the price of $1.00 drew me toward the dismembered tree. I was so fortunate that I still had a little bit of baby-sitting money. I was also fortunate that the yard sale with its precious box was only a block from my home, well within the dragging ability of my 15-year-old self. The only problem was that buying this tree would be an act of defiance.

The last time we had a Christmas tree and celebrated Christmas in my home I had been five years old. That was the last time our family had any extra money. I remember my mother giving me a Teddy bear that year and telling me wistfully that she would never be able to afford another gift so grand. As the years passed and bills were often left unpaid, celebrating was an extravagance that we could not afford. So rather than take handouts or charity, my Father forbade much celebration of the blessed day. He would let Mom make a nice meal if she did not have to work on Christmas. He would let us visit our Aunt Minnie and Aunt Hilda's houses and celebrate there in the days after Christmas, but there was to be no Christmas tree in our house.

I paid the nice lady at the church yard sale my dollar; she even threw a few ornaments in with the purchase. I hefted the unwieldy box and carried it home. Our house door was a bit of a challenge to navigate with the heavy box, but I carried it through the living room and into my bedroom.

Once in my bedroom, I dumped the contents upon the floor. The tree was a post with many small holes and the evergreen branches had colors coded on each twisted metal end. It took a while to figure out the coding system but soon I had a somewhat crooked tree with smattering of ornaments.

With the rest of my babysitting money I bought items at the dime store that I could afford for my family. My mother would get a new coin purse and chocolate covered cherries. I bought my brother Eugene thin mints. The most extravagant gift would go to my sister Esther. I found a wonderful Mickey Mouse doll at the gift shop I knew she would love. I wrapped the gifts and put them underneath the Christmas tree that stood within in my bedroom.

Then I waited.

I waited to see what Dad would do. I waited to see if he would smash it all. I waited to see if he would whip me for my impudence. He looked into my room at the tree. He looked at me. I crossed my arms across my chest and stared at him. He worked his jaws and I saw the anger muscles in his face move threateningly, but he turned and walked away saying "You better keep that in your room, girl."

I sighed with relief and knew I had just witnessed a Christmas miracle.

That Christmas was a slight reprieve in a time of great stress within our family, but in the face of great adversity my defiance would only grow. In the fall of 1989 Dad would threaten to kill us all with the gun I bought in sixth grade. That fall Dad sat at the kitchen table drinking and spinning the gun in lazy circles on the melamine tabletop. My mother washed the dishes at the sink with silent tears running down her cheeks. My sister Esther tried to study. Our adult brother Eugene was living and hiding in his trailer in the backyard. I went back and forth doing the laundry. Dad finally passed out close ten o'clock at night. That was enough. My little sister and I were going to run away.

Esther and I packed two small bags and ran over to Katie and Angie Berg's house. From their house, I called the hotline number I had saved since fourth grade, just in case the abuse became too bad. We were told to go to a local youth shelter. Our friend and fellow student, Robb Fulks, drove us to there.

We went to the shelter and spent almost two weeks at the facility. The staff and volunteers at the shelter were so kind. They helped get a court order preventing our dad from being within 250 feet of us. When I showed signs of anemia, they had me checked at a local hospital. After years as an uninsured child, I was amazed they would have me checked because I "might" have something wrong. In addition, the shelter provided balanced meals that the staff encouraged us to help prepare. I learned more about proper nutrition during mealtimes at the shelter than I had ever learned at home or school.

Although the experience was mostly a good one, there were challenges in shelter life. Esther was very sad with worry that we might be placed in foster care or be sent to live in Enid with our Aunts. She loved her friends and school in Sapulpa and did not want to go. The fellow residents were a mix of children who had been abused and teens that had committed crimes. We bunked in large rooms with several girls in one large space. Esther was a deep sleeper so she did not hear the whispered conversations of our bunkmates, but I did. Late one night two girls planned to ambush the night volunteer and escape. The volunteer was a sweet older lady named Mrs. Humble who had a metal plate in her head and walked with a cane. The girls planned to feign sickness to get her upstairs and then push her down the staircase. I knew that at the volunteer's age and level of physical infirmity, this was likely to kill her. I waited a few moments then ran to the bathroom loudly while inducing vomit. I then excused myself saying I was ill and needed to get some medicine. I went straight to the volunteer and told her of the girls' plan to harm her. Mrs. Humble called the police and the two girls were removed from the shelter. She then hugged me and thanked me, saying that God meant me to be here at this moment so I could help others.

At the end of the two weeks in the shelter, my Mother decided to leave my Father rather than lose her daughters. It was a hard decision, but those two weeks of us away gave her the courage to make that choice. We were so fortunate we had a shelter to go to. We spent the last two years of our youth in a home without the constant threat of violence. Dad realized he needed to get in control of his alcoholism and would end up living for ten more years.

The Christmas tree of 1989 was set up in the living room, and my Mother even set out her fragile Santa mugs so long hidden safely in a box. In the days before Christmas, the doorbell rang. Two strangers stood beneath our threshold with two paper grocery bags filled with wrapped gifts. They were volunteers at the shelter who had heard the testimony I had given against my father. They knew about our years without Christmas.

A Mentor

THE UPHEAVAL IN OUR LIVES in the fall of 1989 did impact our academic lives. Both Esther and I were failing chemistry by mid-fall. We went to the school counselor with our concerns and she said we would be allowed to drop the course with no impact to our GPA. I would be allowed to take double classes of speech and debate and my sister Esther would join us in competitive speaking. Esther was very shy. In some ways she would rather stay in a failing chemistry course than speak publically. I felt so bad for Esther. She was one so nervous that the audience could watch the flush of terror overcome her face. As she would debate in her best church dress a horizontal line of red would creep up her neck toward her face until her cheeks flamed and her voice trembled with fear. I was so proud of her by the spring of 1990. She was an accomplished speaker who qualified for regional competition.

In the spring of 1991, I was a senior year in high school. My sister Esther and I were now very active in speech and debate. My goal was to qualify to attend regional competition in every category of competitive speech. I also hoped to attend national competition. I very nearly reached my goal. I did compete in every category of competitive speech prior to regionals. As a freshman and sophomore I competed in Prose and Standard Oratory, as those categories are exclusive to those years. In the school year of 1990-1991 I competed in

Original Oratory, Dramatic Interpretation, Humorous Interpretation, Domestic Extemporaneous, Foreign Extemporaneous, Monologue, Humorous Duet, Dramatic Duet, and Poetry. I also debated in the Lincoln-Douglas style of debate. I placed among the top three performers in every category at least one time. My sister qualified as well with a lovely original oratory comparing the ups and downs of life within the metaphor of a yo-yo's path.

It was a lot of work, but I am very glad I did it. I memorized hours of material in the attempt. I pored over newspapers and magazines to create files of support documentation for my extemporaneous speech. I spent hours organizing data for quick access when needed. I carried those files in heavy file boxes from tournament to tournament. I had no idea how such preparation would help me in the years to come.

My success was somewhat amazing when one considers our family background. Neither one of my parents had graduated high school. We were very poor. My parents were going through the process of divorce after years of domestic abuse. I had no money for the multiple fine dresses one needed for the competition. Everything was set against me, but I had a special reason for succeeding.

I had a mentor.

Jeanne DeVilliers, otherwise known as "D," was my debate coach. She was a wonderful woman who was there for me in so many ways. She helped me pick out amazing material to perform. She constantly challenged me to do better. Well aware of my history of abuse, she encouraged me to perform a selection from *The Prince of Tides* as a way to work through my angst and use that negative energy toward a positive goal. She would even take me shopping to get the appropriate clothes. I remember her lessons and words to this day. There is not a speech that I perform without feeling her supportive presence.

In 1990, my debate coach recommended me to represent Sapulpa High School at Oklahoma Girl's State. I was going to attend an invitation-only event where most attendees were economically far above my station in life. I was beginning to understand that the individual voice one brings to such an event shines far above any preconceived standing within society. You may be no one of importance when you walk through that door, but the event is created and informed by the voices that attend.

It was spring of 1990. We were still very poor. Both my sister and I worked part-time to pay for our clothes and school extras. Our mother gave us as much as she could, but she was a hospital housekeeper working at minimum wage. Things were tight and we were scraping by. That spring, I was called to the school counselor's office. "You and Heather Pray have been selected to represent Sapulpa High School at Oklahoma Girl's State," the counselor said. I looked at her with surprise as she continued, "Girl's State is a week of student congress hosted at a university. Girls who have good citizenship skills are selected from every high school in the state of Oklahoma to represent their schools. It is an honor to be selected."

I left the counselors office filled with joy, clutching the registration paperwork in my hands. Girl's State! I was so happy, but then I began to read the papers and grew concerned. How could I afford to go? I would need to find transportation to a university many miles away, and according to the paper work I would need a wardrobe consisting of 7 different dresses. Girls wore dresses all week at Girl State.

I had been in Speech and Debate for a year so I owned two performance dresses. Our family attended church, so I had a very nice church dress. I could not afford to go shopping for more. What would I do? I was feeling very like Meg in *Little Women* with no gown for the ball. Fortunately, I was blessed and several of my friends offered to let me borrow their best outfits. Heather Pray and her parents offered to transport us to the college for the week.

All the economic barriers were surmounted! I was going to Girl's State!

It was quite the culture shock when I got there. Most of the ladies running Girl State had been part of sororities and we were taught an equal mix of student government and etiquette; such as the proper way to sit and place one's feet while seated on a dais in a dress. We were also taught quite a few songs that felt straight out of the 1950s such as *"You got to be a Girl State Gal to Amount to Anything!"* and *"A Boy and A Girl In a Little Canoe."* The mornings were filled with pep assemblies with campfire songs and the afternoons were lessons in government. In order to learn about the political process, we created a two party system: the Boomer party and the Sooner party. Soon campaigning began for Sooner and Boomer candidates for governor.

I decided to run. With the help of my campaign manager Jammie Kimmel from Lawton, Oklahoma, I won the Sooner party nomination for governor. We then began the fierce campaign of trying to win governor of Girl's State. We made campaign posters until late into the night. Things were going well and then the time came for a debate in front of hundreds of girls. I had never presented before so many people in my life. I remember staring into the endless crowd as I answered policy question after policy question. This would be the deciding debate. Then they asked the hardest question of them all: "What is your stance on abortion?"

I paused for a few seconds, while thoughts roared within my mind. Time spun through years of my life. I was a girl who could not afford to be here, wearing borrowed dresses. I was a child who had never had insurance coverage and dreaded every sickness. I was a daughter who fought off rape in elementary school. My heart swelled within my chest and I answered: "Regardless, of what I would choose to do within my own personal life, I firmly support the right of a woman to choose medically what happens to her own body." It seemed the silence that followed lasted for years as blood rushed within my ears.

I lost the race for the governor, but I had discovered something very important about myself. No matter what the venue, I would be true to my beliefs in supporting rights of those who are oppressed. I would represent the poor and the abused.

I was a very good student at Sapulpa High School, but I was twice sent to the principal's office. I was sent once for health and once for comedy. I was a journalist for the high school newspaper and was looking for a story. The student body had recently completed a survey wellness check. I found out the school office had a copy of the results. I wrote an article reporting the findings. The statistics I mentioned included drug use, alcohol use, and sexual promiscuity within the school. After turning in my story, I received a summons from the principal. The school paper would not print my story. I wondered aloud if I had made a mistake in my fact checking. The answer was no--they just did not want me to expose the results of the wellness check.

In the spring of 1991, I wrote and directed the senior assembly, including the skits. I was called to the office yet again, as some of the skits contained a comedic analysis of the school that was a bit too scathing. I was ordered to revise the skits and make them "nice." I to some extent complied, although a little of the original biting humor remained. I was tired of being called to the principal's office. I thought it was rather ironic that it was called the principal's office, as I found my principles tended to get trampled there.

Also that spring, I qualified in regional competition and attended the Oklahoma 1991 4a State Competition in both Original Oratory and Poetry. After many grueling rounds in both events, I won state Champion in Poetry recitation. I had performed *The First Quarrel* by Alfred Lord Tennyson. It is a heart--wrenching poem about the last harsh words between a husband and wife before the husband is lost at sea. I was honored to win the State Championship in poetry, but the greatest event was yet to come. Regional competitions can take you to state, but National Forensic League district competition can take you to nationals.

I was so excited to attend district competition.

Many speakers would disdain the judges at regular competitions. At simple qualifying regional events judges were often regular people: bus drivers and locals that wanted to get the twenty-dollar payment for judging for the day. Their only instructions were the rules on the top of the ballot. They would judge for or against based on simple things like whether you were persuasive or not. They wouldn't notice whether you were completely correct in your citations. They did not realize the great error of gesturing too much in poetry or moving both feet in dramatic interpretation. Bus drivers and locals tended to focus on performance and not rules or points or citations. I loved them. There were no power plays and no infighting. They often gave me ballots with the most worthwhile instruction.

At district competition, every judge was immensely qualified. They were all coaches or prior students now pursing college degrees. They were all very aware of the rules and following breakout sheets just like a basketball fan follows the brackets during March Madness. I was so excited during the breakout postings as my name kept rising on the lists, until at last I was in final competition in two events. I competed in both dramatic interpretation and original oratory.

Due to a failure of communication, I was judged down in both.

Prior to the announcement of the winners, my wonderful coach Jeanne DeVilliers took me aside. She said, "Sweetie, I have some bad news for you." I looked at her in horror. I looked at the thin translucent skin of her face, her sparse eyelashes and her carmine lips. I really did not want to look in her understanding eyes as she told me what had happened. I had been in two finals rounds. Each round had three judges. Those two sets of the three judges had not spoken to each other, but both sets had made a fatal error as far as my national competition hopes were concerned. Both sets of very qualified judges had judged against my performance in an attempt to give more seniors the chance to attend nationals. They had both assumed I would come in first or second in the other competition, and so accordingly, both sets of judges had judged me in third place.

I failed to qualify for Nationals. I would not get to speak in Washington DC. It might not seem like a very big deal. But to me it seemed as though my world had crashed down around me. For a very long time, this was the worst moment in my academic life. I was a failure. I would go to college in the fall, still thinking I was a failure.

Broken Trust

In 1991, Esther and I enrolled in college courses at Oklahoma State University. My mother drove us to Bennett dorm in her ancient Impala as neither Esther nor I drove a car. She seemed to feel very uncomfortable on the college campus and left after helping us unload. She said she would see us again at Thanksgiving. Esther quickly assimilated to the college life, much as she had done in elementary school and high school. I began to feel set adrift.

I had followed my boyfriend from my senior year in high school to this university. I would have been a better fit for a small art school rather than a sprawling campus with thousands of students. I rapidly began to feel lost within the masses of students who were all successful. Within weeks of the semester beginning, my boyfriend told me he was breaking up with me. He told me he was actually gay. He also confessed he had cheated on me with most of my male friends.

I broke.

I had been through too much. Too many years of being strong crumbled around me as I processed the truth that what I thought was love was all a lie. It would take me many years to forgive him. As I grew in wisdom as an adult, I realized I was partially at fault. I had attended two different high school proms with two different men and both turned out to be gay. Most of my close male friends were gay. I had spent so much of my youth hiding from the dangers of sexuality that it had become a state of being. I was still hiding as an adult.

I poured all my sorrow into art and theatre. I was cast in a main stage production of the Sam Shepard play *Buried Child*. If you have not had the honor of seeing a production of this piece of art, you may not know that it is really messed up. The director believed in method acting, so he did his utmost best to mess with our minds. The dirty junk-filled set, nonsensical plot, and general unease of the piece was off putting to most of the cast. I felt at home within the cacophony. The set design was sublime. It reflected well the madness of the family that resided within. I played the character of Shelly. She was metaphorically raped on stage, was potentially not real, and was slowly disappearing from the plot. I began to really identify with Shelly.

Time management was a big problem for me throughout this year. Each day I would rehearse the current play and each night I would paint and build the sets. I was so tired. I would try to attend classes and work at my part time job in the library bindery. I fell behind in my classes endangering both my scholarships and my federal grants. Like my father, I turned to alcohol to deaden the pain of life. The alcohol only made my depression worsen. I lost a lot of weight. My fellow actors in turn scorned me or were concerned about my sanity. Esther and her friends came to every play and often brought me flowers. Even with my sister's help, I barely managed to finish the spring semester. Esther was thriving and would decide to spend the summer in Stillwater with her new best friend and roommate. In May I could not wait to return home to my Mom.

I was 20 years old that summer. I spent the warm summer days with my mother in the house I lived in as a child. I had only been away for less than a year. It had been a very hard year. I felt so alone. I was not doing very well in college. I was falling. I was failing. I went home to my mother's embrace, but I was unable to sit still for long.

Soon I was volunteering for the local community theatre. I only had one year of college but that was deemed sufficient training to be in charge of costume design and stage construction for the community theatre production of *Oliver*. Every spare moment I was building costumes or building sets on the local high school stage. I scheduled a work call and only one person showed up to help. Fortunately he was a contractor, so we got quite a bit done. The next day I began hauling fifty-pound drums of drywall mud to the set, when I felt my back go out. Once I could breathe through the pain I went to the office and called my Mom. She came in her car to get me. I could barely walk. Going to the doctor was out of the question since we had no insurance, so she placed me on her bed to rest with an ice pack on my back. She rolled me over as needed, because I could not do that myself.

I lay within the room upon the softest white sheets. In the center of the sheet my mother had embroidered a peacock in a sacred tone of blue. I would run my hands over the hundreds of French knots that marked the plumage. An occasional gentle breeze would blow in from the open window and the window sheers would billow like the wings of angel. My mother cared for me. Soon the show's director called. She wanted me to come in and work on the set. My Mother is the sweetest, kindest person you could ever meet. I had never seen her raise her voice outside the family. But that night she yelled on the phone at the director of the show, and I smiled. I knew my mother had my back, even if I had broken it.

The Cleaning Of The Brush

IN THE FALL OF 1992, I went back to college. I went back because that is
what is expected. I went back because my best friend from high school,
T.J Jones, was now a freshman and we wanted to get an apartment together. My back was better, but my mind was not. I continued to build
sets and to paint scenery, but I was no longer cast main-stage produc-
tions. The professors had placed me on academic probation based on
my poor grades in any class that was not theatre. I had very little money
and what little I had I gave to my best friend to cover rent.

When my future husband, Fred, saw me for the first time, I was painting. I was painting letters on a theatre drop curtain. My hair hung long
within a braid. I was kneeling brush in hand. I did not see him standing
in the fly-space looking down upon me. The first time we ever talked,
we stood in front of the old soda machine in the Green Room at OSU.
As the old machine hummed its refrigerated whine, I sipped Mountain
Dew and spoke of Randal Flag. Fred looked at me with golden-flecked
blue eyes and quoted *The Dark Tower* back to me.

I officially met Frederick Allen Holliday II, in scenic painting class.
He was taking the class for graduate credit. He could take either costume construction or scenic painting. He thought painting would be
easier. I remember him using the words "blow off" class. I was a second

year freshman barely passing my classes, but pretty good at painting, so I enrolled in it as well. Every week we each painted a 5'x5' canvas. I taught him how to clean his brushes in the deep sinks and helped him prepare his palette. The rest of the class would come and go every day and get their paintings done gradually. Fred and I both liked to procrastinate. Each week we would show up at nine or ten. We would paint all night. I got to know Fred by pulling all-nighters with him for months. There is no better way to get to know the real person than pulling routine all-nighters.

Have you ever pulled an all-nighter? You weren't exactly chipper and bright were you? Fred would show up dressed in Metallica sweat pants. He would be wearing an Anthrax t-shirt under a magenta dress shirt. The ubiquitous walk-man tape player would dangle from his pocket. He listened to his hard rock music so loud I could hear it from ten feet away. I would paint silently. He would go on and on about news from *Entertainment Weekly* and *Premiere*. I would paint silently. He would frantically gesticulate while painting and quote the entire movie *Star Wars* from memory. I finally set my brush down and said in my most put-upon voice, "You are a walking advertisement for the entertainment industry!" He looked at me with his infuriating smile and upraised eyebrow said, "I take that as a compliment." Back to work he went with a jaunty step and that silly smile. I was furious.

I threw a sponge at him. He got rather wet and I smiled. A little later he came over to me with a can of Pepsi and poured liquid all over my head. I could not believe he drenched me in soda! (It turns out he didn't. He had replaced the soda with cold water, but wasn't going to tell me.) I was doubly furious. It was full on wet sponge war at three in the morning on the main stage. We finished our rather splotchy paintings and went our separate ways for about thirty minutes as we had class at 8:00 am. Any third grader could have told us that we were beginning to fall in love.

We finished the semester and went to our homes for Christmas. After a few days without Fred, I missed our fights. I did not know that Fred was missing me too. Fred was very homesick for Maryland and I was not sure he really wanted to be in Oklahoma. As the winter break came to a close, I went back to Stillwater to stay with T.J in our apartment. Money was getting really tight. T.J's fiancé Evan suggested we consider joining the military. I started to seriously look at the Navy.

Throughout the rest of the winter break, I was spending hour upon hour playing hearts with T. J and her fiancée, Evan. I was often a cautious player, but when the deck was stacked against me and my back was against the wall, I would "Shoot the Moon." I would either win the hand or fail miserably. There was no in between.

At that time in my life I was only 20. I was preparing to join the Navy and had not yet kissed a man named Fred Holliday II. He was only 22 years old himself. I was having trouble paying rent and was most definitely following the path of many an artist and theatre major, by failing half of my college classes.

My life was at a crossroads. I would have to make a fateful decision, to fold my hand or to "Shoot the Moon." During this time of stress, I walked the path of my father and wrote quite a bit of poetry. I wrote the poem below during this period.

Hearts

Though darkness is spreading all over my land,
The cards, they still could lie.
The Black Sister hides her face this night,
Not yet my time to die,
At least not with these hearts in my hand.

~Regina Hollliday

I called Fred when he was back from break. I asked him if he would go with me to a theatre party. He said, "Sure, I will drive you. I know you don't have a car." The minute we got to the party he went in the other room with the guys and talked about *The Godfather* films. The party host played dance music. I asked Fred to dance. He replied, "I don't dance." I was running out of ideas of how to ascertain if Fred liked me. Fred asked me if I would like to see the movie *The Fisher King* at his place. I said emphatically, "Yes!" We went to his place and *began to watch the movie*. He started to tell me all about the actors and the director. He was talking a mile a minute. I kissed him. Finally, he got the hint.

I started dating Fred at the same time I was going through the recruiting process to join the Navy. Within two months I was engaged to Fred, yet I still planned to go to boot camp in May immediately after my 21st birthday. Fred left Oklahoma State and enrolled in a graduate program at American University in Washington, DC. Fred moved back to Maryland for the summer as I took my first airplane ride to Florida. I made it through boot camp in Orlando, even running a mile and a half on a knee with torn ligaments. On a sunny day in July, I graduated from boot camp. I was so proud to wear my dress whites on the parade field in Orlando. Then I spent two glorious weeks with Fred on leave before going to technical school in Chicago. I even painted a mural in the local Navy recruiting office in Cumberland, Maryland. The officers loved that painting so much. Several years later when they moved their offices they sawed through the drywall and took the painting with them. I received a commendation for the work. Then I left for technical school and darkness descended.

Both Fred and I sank deep into depression in our lonely rooms so far apart. I did not want to fail again. I did not want to fail in technical school. I did not want to fail in love. I was bunking alone in a strange city. I knew almost no one in Chicago. I was spiraling into sadness. I wanted to stick it out and succeed in the Navy, but that wasn't in the cards. So, I folded. During this dark time, I was admitted into the Naval hospital for psychiatric treatment. I didn't take medication for my depression. I just talked with the counselors and I drew. I find art to be an amazing form of treatment.

I began a very large pencil drawing. The staff said it was a nice picture, but why the really big empty space? I explained that it was my life story, and my life was far from over. I think that was the right answer, because I was soon released. I left with an entry-level separation for situational depression. I never wore my dress whites again. I traded them for a white gown. I decided to play the hand I was dealt with a man who loved me as much as I loved him and with whom I could not live without. I felt guilty about leaving the Navy for a very long time. I hope in some small measure my work to improve health care for us all in the years hence, make up in part for having to separate from the armed forces.

From October through December of 1993, I would live with my mother, brother and Grandfather again. I would help my old debate coach at the high school prepare a new group of eager students for their regional competition and I would slowly rebuild my heart and mind. Fred and I would call each other at least once a week. We would write long love letters to each other and I would write him poems on my ancient typewriter. We would marry very soon and I wanted him to know I took that "till death do us part" oath very seriously. I wrote him this poem in November of 1993:

Not I Amongst the Rows

They say someday they'll bury me
But I ask of he who marries me
As he still lives and surely knows
Not I amongst the rose.

Though the posy may hold sway
And roses pave the passage way
Pray don't lay me down to rest
Weighted garlands on my chest.

But if they must bequeath the dead
With leafy greens and flower beds
Well, tear mine up, hack and hack
To mulch the cactus on my back.

I guess I'm quite a rarity
Yearning now for liberty.
Formless? Not I, instead
Standing out amongst the dead.

A bridge I'd want for monument
A path to me it represents
A road to he who called me wife
The reason why I lived my life.

Plant the cactus all around
For beauty grows in arid ground
And blooms so pretty in the night
As did our love in life's twilight.

Tend my grave as though I'm there
Say sweet nothings in the air
But never pull a single weed
let them grow and let them seed.

Let nature reign the place I left
And leave no plot for the bereft
I'll have no one buried near
Except for he who was most dear.

They say someday they'll bury me
But I ask of he who marries me
As he still lives and surely knows,
Not I amongst the rows.

No green grown mediocrity
No rows of uniformity
Another daisy in another bed
Plant me not in groves of dead.

Mark me not in stone to stay
As though a fact to file away
Memory of me live or die
But far away in some mind's eye.

I have learned, no one's to blame
All the dangers of the same
I have won my sanity
But know with equal certainty

Stack me not head to toe
Ask me not to file in row
As he still lives and surely knows
Not I amongst the rose.

Our wedding was on December 26, 1993 in Enid, Oklahoma. Fred's parents, Fred and Joan Holliday, drove with him all the way from Maryland to take part in the wedding. Fred and I were so poor. I sold all my comic books to pay for the wedding invitations, and Fred sold all of his comic books to pay for our rings. (He was a DC fan and I was Marvel fan so it was the best choice for marital peace.) I wore my mother's wedding dress and my grandmother's veil. Fred wore a nice suit. Poinsettias were the wedding flowers as Immanuel Lutheran Church was already decorated for Christmas. Our groomsmen wore suits and our bridesmaids wore church dresses. It was a beautiful wedding.

Our First Home

THE DAY AFTER OUR WEDDING, we loaded up my father-in-law's truck with my scant possessions and I left Oklahoma and moved to Grantsville, Maryland. My mother-in-law, Joan, and my father-in-law, Fred, were very kind. They took me in as Fred was living in the dorms at American University at the time, and I could not live with him for our first five months of marriage.

This was a very unusual experience for me. Fred Senior was a loving father and upstanding citizen. I was not used to being around a supportive father figure. Fred Sr. was very involved in the local community and was the mayor of the town of Grantsville from 1983-1998. He ran the local hardware store and the family residence was right above the store. Even after hours, Fred would open up the store and help local folks out in an emergency. Joan was an adoring mother to my Fred. She called her son everyday and Fred would call her back. They loved each other very much. Joan was a secretary at Frostburg State University 1963-1969, and then she quit to have little Fred. She stayed home with him and his two adopted sisters until 1981. That year she went back to work at Frostburg State as a secretary in the Theatre Department. She would work there until 2007. She was loved by all the students and acted as a substitute mom for many far from home. Each morning that winter Joan would get up very early to safely traverse the snowy roads from Grantsville to Frostburg.

Grantsville is a lovely small town built in the foothills of the Appalachian Mountains. Here it began to snow in January and did not stop till April. I had never been so cold in all of my life. Within a few weeks of arriving I began working in the local Flushing Shirt Factory. I had never had a factory job before. It was hard, dirty work. I operated the inking plate that labeled shirts with their material content. The type was old, worn, and needed frequent cleaning with caustic chemicals that would burn through my work gloves on a fairly regular basis. When I left work, I would walk to my in-laws house trudging through snowdrifts. Some days were so cold I could feel ice form in my eyelashes as my glasses frosted over. I could not see the leaves on the trees, as there were no leaves, just an endless expanse of snow.

In the fall of 1994, Fred and I leased the cheapest apartment we could find in DC. We finally had our own place. The apartment was the upstairs floor of a house belonging to an elderly woman who was retired CIA. She drank like a sailor and smoked like a chimney. Each week the liquor store would deliver a case of vodka to the front door. Our landlady was also very hard of hearing but told the most amazing stories. Of course she said she could not tell all of her stories, as they were still top secret.

I began to look for a job. I worked briefly at the Foreign Service Club as the dessert girl. Fred was very focused on school and was not sure he could commit to a part time job. I looked at the money I had saved from working six months at the shirt factory rapidly disappearing in this costly new city and told Fred we both had to work to make ends meet. I opened the paper and showed him an advertisement for a job at a toy store really close to our apartment.

That store was Barston's Child's Play, and Fred was immediately hired. New employees at that store must attend a game night so they can learn how to play the games. Spouses are invited, so Fred and

I went to play with Fred's employer, Steven and his wife, Simmie. I am a very competitive player so I rapidly went from being a pleasant quiet wife to doing everything I could to beat my husband's new boss. Within a few weeks, I was hired too. After a few months, I was an assistant manager in one of the best toys stores in our nation's capital. Fred and I worked side by side for many months, but soon the video store next door was hiring and Fred thought that would be a better job choice based on his interest in film and his encyclopedic knowledge of the genre.

Within six months of being hired at the toy store, Steven gave me a form to fill out for health insurance. I read the questions on it. "Were you hospitalized in the last five years? And if so where and for what reason?" I was terrified and embarrassed. I knew I could not fill out that form and turn it in. I would have to admit to hospitalization in a psychiatric facility only a year before and I was sure that could cost me this job. I told my boss I was turning down the insurance. He looked at me quizzically, "You understand that we pay for it, it won't come out of your salary." I still shook my head no. He continued, "If you don't come aboard now you will not be eligible for another year…" I still said no, I did not want it. He walked away shaking his head. In 1995, 1996, & 1997 I would be given the form again. Each time I would turn down the insurance after reading, "Were you hospitalized in the last five years?" With wisdom and age, I know now that I could have told Steven and he would have understood, but then I was too frightened.

I cherished the many years I worked at Child's Play. I learned so much about toys and child development. Steven was always lending us books so we could be experts on the sales floor. Occupational therapists, speech language therapists, and child psychologists used a lot of our toys. Many of these professionals referred parents to our store. We would also get referrals from local private schools and testing services. We helped customers in the moments after they had been given the devastating news that their child has a learning disability, sensory integration dysfunction, or autism.

We would gently show them potential choices that might help with therapeutic play. During these consultations, I often helped a customer for over an hour even though they would only buy a few items. The parent needed the conversation more than the toy itself. It was hard but it so worth it. It was an honor to help people at such a point in their lives. Sometimes no one told the parent why he or she was sent to buy such toys. Sometimes we would have a hard conversation.

I will never forget the day I helped a young mother. She came in with a list of toys to help practice for a test to get into a new school. I began to ask her what she meant by practice. She informed me that her child had been tested so he could get into a private elementary school. The testing proctor said his scores were "scattered." The child could try again in two years, and meanwhile he could practice. I looked upon the list of toys. It was a prodigious purchase.

If she bought it all, the sale would total well over $500.00 dollars. My eyes scanned the list again, and I grew concerned. This wasn't a prep list for the child of an over-achieving parent.

This was a very specific list. Then I began to ask questions. "When your child was small did he spin wheels?" She nodded her head. "Did he talk early or was it a little later?" "Later," she said. "Did he or does he still have an interest in just one topic like trains, insects or dinosaurs?" She smiled at me and nervously nodded, "Yes! He loves trains and talks about them all the time. He has for years and he has every Thomas the Tank Engine train ever made." I looked down at the list again, took a deep breath and then looked into her eyes. We seemed frozen in a moment, balanced on a tipping point. Her eyes were brimming with emotion, and the tears were held at bay because I had not asked the final question.

"Do you think your child might have autism?"

Then the floodgates opened and she began to cry. "Oh, I do. I do, "she sobbed. "But no one ever says it. What will we do?" I held her hand. I did not sell a lot of products that day, but that was not important. It was more important to help this lovely woman and to have the hard conversation that she had been denied.

If you walk into Child's Play, within moments you are greeted. If you do not immediately ask for help and receive guidance, you will subsequently be asked by every other staff member if you would like help or if you are finding things all right. We will guide you through the entire store showing age appropriate choices with honesty and candor. We will wrap your presents at no charge and help you carry your large purchases to your car. I am glad I got a chance to work at Child's Play off and on since 1994. That experience reminds me that the high bar I have set on patient centered care within the world of medicine is attainable.

Kansas

IN 1997 FRED ENROLLED IN the University of Kansas in the film Department pursuing a doctorate in film studies. We packed our little car and moved to Lawrence, Kansas.

I was hired as the art department manager of the Jayhawk Bookstore in Lawrence. I learned the college book business under the tutelage of Bill Muggy. Bill had been working in the world of college books for over 20 years. He did a little of everything at the store. He ordered some products, created advertisements, and was always looking for the next fad or hook that would engage the public and remind them to shop at our store. That is how I met Nathan Muggy, Bill's son. Nathan was in his early twenties and was a quiet and introspective artist. He would occasionally work at the store, but he would not stay long. Often Bill would bring him in to work on ad copy or during book rush.

In 1997 the catch phrase was *Titanic's* "I am king of the world!" or "You killed Kenny." Every child was begging for a razor scooter and folks were starting to choose that new-fangled Google as their preferred web browser. In the fall of 1997 the newest trend was *South Park*. Bill decided to connect with the incoming youth using this new animation style. So Nathan labored long hours creating a commercial short for the store in the *South Park* Style. As I enjoyed both art and *South Park*, Nathan and I talked quite a bit. After about two weeks Nathan finished the animation work and was gone again. Then Bill purchased an amazing quantity of *South Park* Shirts at the NACS (National Association of College Stores) conference that spring. Jayhawk bookstore was very good at selling Jayhawk merchandise, but we were not famous for trendy fashion choices. So we sold some of those shirts in 1998. By 1999 the gift department staff were eager to place them on the clearance rack.

Then In 1999 Nathan Muggy died.

Bill called me in the early morning that spring day. He said that Nathan had been in an automobile and drove off the side of a mountain. Nathan had hit his head. All of this had happened in the Virgin Islands and Bill would have to fly there later that day to help his son. When Bill arrived Nathan was unconscious and badly injured. His brain was swelling. Nathan lingered for a few days. When it looked like death was inevitable, Bill tried to organize an organ donation team so that Nathan's death would not be in vain. They were not prepared for such requests at the remote hospital, and Nathan died without being a donor as he had wished. In 2000, we placed the last of the South Park Shirts on sale, and I cried. I cried that those shirts were still there and Nathan was not.

We participated in two art shows that year in honor of Nathan Muggy and his art. One of those shows was the *Lawrence Art Walk*. We created a prominent display of Nathan's work from his years in college inside the Jayhawk Bookstore. It was a beautiful dedication. As a thank you for my work honoring Nathan's memory, Bill gave me several of Nathan's paintbrushes. I still paint with them, and in this way Nathan's work lives on.

The other art festival we participated in was *Harvest of the Arts*. This event was organized by one of Fred's students named Lissa Probus. She thought it was lovely that we were honoring Nathan but she wanted to see my paintings too. Fred had explained to the entire class that we had fallen in love painting, and Lissa wanted to see my work. That was going to be hard to do, as I had not painted in five years. I was really busy working. I just did not have time to paint.

Our lives changed a great deal while in Kansas. When we moved to Lawrence, we were still a relatively young couple. We loaded all of our possessions into our tiny car in DC. Then we drove across the country. When saw the cinderblock expanse of married student housing, we quickly realized our bedroom window faced the parking lot but our front door was 100 yards away. We gleefully unloaded a car filled with books, linens, and clothes through that small bedroom window. We slept on the floor that first night, as we hadn't any furniture. I remember the room did not feel empty as we lay there watching the occasional headlight beam illuminate the wall. We held hands across the cool linoleum. We talked till late in the night buoyed by hopes and dreams. In Kansas, we felt the mantle of adulthood firmly embrace us. It was time grow.

We decided to become parents. I took a class with Fred once again. These were Lamaze classes. Each session I would lean back into his warm torso. I placed my hands upon my taunt belly and took a deep breath. I felt the breath deep within, centering me, supporting me. Then I let it go. I was preparing for the time to come: birth, new life and the pain of it all. The instructor said concentrate on the breathing. My body had changed so much. My torso swelled, I was retaining water and could no longer see my ankles. Walking was hard, breathing was hard, but through it all Fred stood beside me.

When Lamaze class ended, the gaggle of pregnant women and the cluster of husbands would mutter in an excited anticipatory way. We were walking this path together and everyone could relate. I read pamphlets and books that would cover every detail of this exciting adventure. I was familiar with terms like contractions, dilated, and active labor. If I tired of reading, I could question our Lamaze instructor or my OBGYN. I could ask my neighbors, friends, and relatives about their birth experience. I didn't even have to ask, folks constantly would tell me their stories un-solicited. We planned the natural birth of our first son. Little Freddie came one month early so we missed the final Lamaze class, but we had learned enough. When labor came Fred held my hand and we breathed together. He looked deep into my eyes and we breathed through the pain. He smiled at me and said, "There see, it is not so hard, just take a deep breath and let it out." I delivered Freddie in September of 1998 by natural childbirth. The lovely doctors and nurses at the hospital were in complete support of my decision. The OB was very excited because this happened so rarely. After his birth Freddie couldn't regulate his temper-ature and had trouble breathing due to his immature lungs. He had to be placed in an incubator. I was very fortunate that I had chosen a natural childbirth. Just hours after delivering Freddie, I could sit by his side in the small NICU. Lawrence Memorial had a very special program for mothers of sick babies. There was a room called the Segebrecht Room, in honor of Dr. Segebrecht, his wife, and their baby, where mothers could stay post discharge and care for compromised infants. I stayed there for a week while Freddie stabilized, and then we went home to our tiny apartment.

Life was very challenging with a new baby. I went back to work with-in 6 weeks as we needed my income and there wasn't any paid maternity leave. Fred's graduate teaching provided a lot of teaching experience but not much income. We were very challenged to find a sitter. We final-ly found one and she watched Freddie for five months. Then we learned that she took summers off. I went to my boss Bill at the bookstore and told him about my dilemma. Bill had seen me backpack Freddie on my days off. We talked about a novel concept that would enable me to work and care for Freddie at the same time. I would backpack Freddie all summer while working. I thought the Native Americans had done this for centuries, surely it would not be so hard.

It was lovely having my son at work, but it was stressful. I worried that the students and professors would find me unprofessional. It was hard on my back and hips, and by July I did need to visit a chiropractor. But I loved the smell of baby Freddie so close to me. I loved the way the college students would change their demeanor and resist using foul language as little Freddie peered at them from over my shoulder. By the fall we found a daycare for Freddie, and I was the acting store manager at the Jayhawk Bookstore. My workload was immense. Fred was teaching classes while taking courses for his doctorate. I was working about 55 hours a week at the store, responsible for the housework and childcare whenever I was home. To this already burdened schedule, Lissa from *Harvest of the Arts* wanted to add a painting.

Life can get in the way of passion. We can always come up with excuses as to why we miss church, can't volunteer, and are too busy to help our friends. I decided to paint a painting even though I was too busy, because it was the right thing to do. When I was in college I wrote a poem called *Genisis 1:8*. The poem was based on a story our Rabbi professor told us about the book of Genesis. He told us in the Talmud there were theologians who thought Genesis is made of multiple stories. One of those stories is the concept that God destroyed the world many times at the urging of his angels because ultimately humanity failed. The theory was that we are living in the world that God did not abort. He kept us even with our blemish. I thought this was an intense poem, but would be even more powerful coupled with a painting.

I painted a picture that I call "The Lady." It depicts a very pregnant woman of indiscriminate race. She represents God and is framed by the Star of David, which is placed upon the darkness of space. The Star of David is made up multicolored rice paper that has the words of the poem inscribed. On both sides of her figure the words from the poem are a decoupage on the canvas. I love this painting. It is peaceful and is beautiful.

The scary part came next. I would have to set up in a field as an artist at an arts festival. Although I have created art all of my life, I have often felt ostracized from the greater arts community. In college, I tried to take a class in the art department, but was told my folk art style and the painting techniques I used in theatre had ruined me for "real art." I had worked for many years selling art supplies at both the toy store and the bookstore, so some in the arts community considered me a "sell out." When I arrived at the field of the art festival, I felt so very small. The other artists had big white tents, numerous paintings and hundreds of cellophane wrapped prints. I stood beside a folding chair that I was using to prop up my 4'x4' painting.

I stood for hours as the sun burned my skin. Few people stopped to talk with me. Why would they? I was a pretty sorry example of an artist with only one painting to my name. I was thankful the sunburn on my cheeks camouflaged my acute embarrassment. Then a woman who looked a few months pregnant walked up to my painting. She stared at it and read the poem in its entirety. Silent tears ran down her face. A muffled sob escaped her lips. Then with her head down she began to speak, "I was just at the doctor's office. He had the results of my test. There is something wrong with my baby. He said I would have to decide what to do. He left me alone to think about it. I had to leave, but I couldn't go home. Not now, not with this. I saw this park. I saw the tents and the flags. I thought I would go there. I will be with people." She looked up at me. Her blue eyes were fierce within their cascade of tears. She said to me, "I came here. I read your poem and saw your painting. I know what to do. I will keep it. I love my baby, even if there is something wrong, I still love my baby." I reached out and embraced her. We cried together.

Moments later she walked away. I never learned her name and I never saw her again. I folded up my chair and carried it with one arm as I hefted my painting with the other. The festival was not over, but I was finished. I had painted that painting for one person in this world and she had seen it. In the worst moment in her life, art was there to help her, just as it had helped me.

There Is Paint In The Oven

As a child, I often drew spirals. I felt at peace when the pencil lead would score the page and the circle turned ever inward. As I grew older, I drew tornadoes, which are just spirals viewed from the side. As an adult, I learned that the Celtic triple spiral represented time, life, and three phases of a woman. But whenever I want to connect with that inner vortex from whence art and love can flow, I start with spirals. When you live within spirals you double back.

In 2001, our family left Lawrence, Kansas and returned to Washington, DC. I would again work at the toy store, and Fred would again work at the video store. Fred had finished his course work and was beginning his dissertation. I was so happy to return to the toy store, and this time when Steven handed me the paperwork for insurance I said, "Yes, I want it." I had no idea how hard it would be to find a primary care doctor in DC who was still accepting patients. I called page after page of doctors in my insurance directory. I was told again and again we are not accepting new patients. Finally I found an office nearby willing to see me. When I arrived the waiting room was filled with patients with white or silver hair. I waited my turn to see the doctor. When the doctor entered the exam room and he smiled. He said, "You are Regina?" I said yes. He smiled a bit more and said, "You are a bit younger than the majority of my patients. My specialty is geriatrics." I was crestfallen. I asked, "Does that mean you cannot be my doctor?" He said, " Oh I can be your doctor but you may be one of my younger patients." He would be my doctor for the next eight years.

Time went by fast in DC. Fred was writing his dissertation based on the long narrative in *Buffy The Vampire Slayer* (1997-2003). Our little son Freddie was enrolled in the local private preschool CCBC (Chevy Chase Bethesda Community Children's Center). After volunteering as a parent at my son's children's center for a year, I proposed to the Director that they hire me to teach art. I began working there two days a week whilst working five days a week at Child's Play. For the next few years I would have very few days off.

I loved helping children and their families with art. At the toy store students or parents would come into my art section and say, "Please help me!" A project would be due within hours and the customer would need my expert advice on how to finish or salvage their work. This was not active art on my part, but I loved helping them I loved building up the work inside my head seeing all the potential pitfalls and helping to avoid them. These customers were frustrated and I was happy to have the chance to help them through art.

As the years passed and word of mouth grew, people would call Child's Play just to ask me about school art projects. My boss, Steven, would show such patience with customers who would talk to me for thirty minutes then buy only a few items and leave. He understood that the customer would remember that we had helped them out in their time of stress. We had listened, asked questions, made eye contact and had given the customer options. After years selling art supplies, I began getting requests to help with auction projects at my son's school as well as schools throughout DC. Most schools in DC have an annual auction in which class creations can raise money for the school. I was sometimes called in to help facilitate this process.

In those days, Fred and I infrequently went on dates or hired baby sitters. Upon the rare occasions we would go out, it was usually to attend a school auction in support of the work of our son and my young art students. Before we would go out, I would place a note on the refrigerator. In addition to the regular emergency numbers and instructions for care, I would write a warning: "There is paint in the oven." As an art teacher living in a series of small, carpeted apartments, there was only one place to paint, in the kitchen. So my counters were covered in brush bins and paint buckets. My sink filled with paint splotches and my kitchen apron is an artist's smock. There was so little space available I could waste none. So when I was not cooking, the oven was a convenient location for paint storage. Fred and I knew to empty it before pre-heating, but I always worried that a babysitter would just cook my paints.

This was a very creative time in many ways. In 2005 Freddie finished his dissertation and was working as an adjunct instructor at Carroll County Community College. We had decided to have a second child. Freddie had been a very challenging young child to raise and was diagnosed with sensory dysfunction and was well on his way to an autism diagnosis. We wanted to make sure he had a sibling while he was still young enough for them to play together. I had been very close to both my brother and sister growing up. Fred was an only child until his sisters were adopted when he was four. We both knew the importance of siblings.

By winter of 2006, I was just trying to maintain my pregnancy. I had begun pre-term labor before Thanksgiving and was carefully watching for further contractions. My OB told me that as long as I drank water constantly and didn't lift anything, I should be able to make it to 36 weeks. I was still working at the toy store but had to stop teaching so I could rest two days out of seven. In late January, I woke to find Freddie sick and I still needed to go to my OB appointment. Fred stayed home with Freddie. I took the bus and then the metro to my appointment, where I was told that I was beginning to dilate but had not dropped. I took the train and the bus back home to find Freddie running a 104-degree temperature. I called the pediatrician to make a sick care appointment. They fit him in that afternoon and told us he had a bad case of the flu. While at that appointment I felt the contractions begin. So we drove across town to the OB, who determined I had dilated quite a bit more, so he recommended I go to the hospital.

In rush hour traffic my worried husband drove me to the hospital with our sick little boy in the back seat. Fred had to deposit me on the curb. I waddled into the hospital by myself and went to stand in the line for submitting insurance information. After triaging me they said my blood pressure was too high to walk around as I had done in my last labor. I was told to lie on a gurney in the labor triage while they waited for a room to open up. After enduring a few hours of ever increasing contractions with no relief via movement or distracting company, I was finally transferred to labor and delivery. I had already made it very clear during the entire process I wanted natural childbirth.

As I labored without my husband or a friend to advocate for me, I saw something out of the corner of my eye. A nurse was doing something. I whipped my head around and asked, "What are you doing to my line?" She looked over at me nonchalantly and said, "I am adding Pitocin to speed up labor." "No, you are not!" I said. "I had my first son in five hours and I will have this one in less and don't you dare touch my line."

She left in huff and I was once again alone in the room. Everything happened very fast after that. Fred finally arrived, as my mother-in-law was able to drive up and watch little Freddie. Within thirty minutes my water broke and we had Isaac. His face crinkled in dismay at being born and Fred immediately said he looked like a little old man. Fred was right. Looking at Isaac was like looking at a miniature version of my father.

They took Isaac to the NICU, but he seemed to be doing pretty well considering he was barely 36 weeks old. Fred looked at me lovingly and said, "I brought you something to read." It was Stephen King's book: *Cell.* I loved that book, and I agreed with its premise that cell phones create zombies. I swore I would never own a cell phone. The next day the NICU staff said they wanted to send Isaac home. He was slightly underweight with an elevated bilirubin. I was very concerned. His brother was holding at 102 degrees and was vomiting. Our tiny one bedroom was completely contaminated. I had not even been allowed home yet to clean. The staff suggested we could always go to a hotel. I walked away and called the pediatrician's office. A couple of hours later the NICU director told me, "I don't know who your pediatrician is but she just tore me a new one. Your son may stay for two days." I checked out and went home. I ate some take-out, expressed some milk and then began disinfecting the apartment, as my mother-in-law, Joan, comforted Freddie. Then Fred went back to work a shift at the video store.

Resolutions

2006 AND 2007 FLEW BY in a rush of work and responsibility. With two children our life became a frantic series of tasks. Baby Isaac was getting into everything. We moved from our more spacious one-bedroom apartment on the eleventh floor to a much smaller one-bedroom on the second floor after eight -year-old Freddie vocalized our inner fears that dare-devil Isaac would somehow fall out the window.

Fred and I were working so many hours. I was teaching at two schools and was working full time at the toy store. In my "free time" I was painting neighborhood murals. Fred was now an adjunct professor at Carroll County Community College, The University of the District of Columbia, and Towson University. He also still pulled shifts at the video store. Even though he was working all the time, he was making very little money, as adjuncts are contract employees without benefits and the video store paid minimum wage. In the 2007/2008 academic school year, I only had four days off: Thanksgiving, Christmas, New Year's Day and Easter. Our schedules were destroying us.

On New Year's Day, Fred and I decided to write down our resolutions for 2008. We knew we would have to change our life path if we were go-ing to survive. Our resolutions were not pie-in-the-sky concepts. They were reasonable life goals:

* Get medical insurance for the whole family.
* Get little Freddie into a special needs school.
* Fred gets a job in his field.
* Spend more time together as a family.
* Get a two-bedroom apartment

Even with our crazy work schedules we could not afford health insurance as a family. I was covered under the toy store policy, but we paid out-of-pocket for Fred and the children. Fred had a pre-existing condition that made a family policy too expensive. We could not afford to pay $1,700.00 each month in rent and pay for a $1,000.00 a month health insurance policy on the open market. We made a little too much money to qualify for poverty care for the children. We were stuck.

Each year Freddie struggled more in public school. He had been on an IEP since kindergarten, but in third grade everything was falling apart. He received a diagnosis of autism and we needed to find a better school setting for him. We retained a wonderful pro bono lawyer and began the process of moving Freddie into a non-public school that focused on autistic children. As there were no schools in DC that specialized in autistic instruction we focused on Ivymount School in Silver Spring, Maryland as a good choice for Freddie.

By 2008, Fred had been in school for most of his adult life. He had completed a Bachelor of Science in Theatre, then a Masters degree and a Doctorate in Film Studies. He had served as a graduate teaching assistant and adjunct professor for many years. He felt he had more than paid his dues and deserved to finally have a job in his field. We would do everything we could to make these resolutions a reality. Our work stress and economic challenges were affecting our family. We wanted to spend more quality time together but not in such close confines. We were a family of four with a rambunctious two-year-old and a nine-year-diagnosed with autism living in a small one-bedroom apartment. Everyone was on edge.

When Fred and I first married, we went on weekly dates. They were wonderful evenings. We would go to a bookstore and each buy a book. Often they would be books by Stephen King. Then we would go to a restaurant and read those books while holding hands. We were so happy that we found each other. We were soul mates. We loved to read together, watched films together and talked with each other till dawn. We married and never stopped talking and were always looking forward to each new Stephen King book. We moved many times in our 15 years of marriage, but the first thing Fred always did was set up his Stephen King shelf of books. I called it the shrine. He loved to show friends and guests these prized books. He said if there ever were a fire the books would leave with him. Fred's house had burned down when he was but thirteen years old: fire was never far from his thoughts. He assured me he would save his books. He said he would also make sure I got out okay afterwards. Then life happened. We had to work and take care of children. There was so little time to read. As the years passed by there was so little time and space just to be together.

In the spring of 2008, Fred and I saw a psychiatrist every week from late January until May. Fred was very depressed, fatigued and was losing weight. Our son had just been officially diagnosed with autism. Fred had taken that rather hard. Fred was also very sad that although he had been an adjunct for years, he could not find a full time job. The psychiatrist was an incredibly nice man who specialized in families with autism. He saw us even though Fred did not have insurance and we would have to pay out-of-pocket. We talked through our problems, and it seemed to help Fred's emotional state. I just wished that he had asked Fred to complete a full physical to rule out an underlying condition for his mental anguish, in addition to providing talk therapy.

We made the most of our weeks of therapy. Fred would pick me up from work during my lunch break. We would hop in our little blue car and drive to the gas station by the doctor's office. There we would park and grab hot dogs, chips, and soda. We would eat on the steps in front of the doctor's office. We called these sessions our "dates." We enjoyed this time with one another just as man and wife, not as Mom and Dad.

That summer Fred was hired by American University as part of the fall faculty. His spirits rose considerably. He was so excited at the age of 38 to finally have a "real job." Dr. Fred Holliday would join the faculty in the fall of 2008 in a split position in the Departments of Literature and Performing Arts, teaching Critical Approach to the Cinema and American Society on Stage and Screen. This new job allowed us to spend more quality time together as a family. The job also came with full benefits, so for the first time everyone in our family had health insurance. Freddie was accepted into Ivymount School for the fall of 2008. Things were looking up!

We still didn't have a two-bedroom apartment, but we thought it was only a matter of time.

Media Still Matters

The Doctor: "You can let me do this."
River Song: "If you die here, it will mean I never met you."
The Doctor: "Time can be re-written!"

River Song: "Not these times. Not one line, don't you dare! It's okay.
It's okay. It's not over for you. You'll see me again. You've got all of
that to come. You and me, time and space; you watch us run."

The Doctor: "River, you know my name. You whispered my name
in my ear. There is only one reason I would ever tell anyone my
name. There is only one time I could."

River Song: "Hush. Shh... now, spoilers."

— *Doctor Who*, 2008, Season 4, episode 9, "Forrest of
the Dead."

Do you paint or draw? When you paint, how do you compose the piece?
There are so many ways to create art. Some artists plan ahead and plot
the course. Then they replicate these designs on a grand scale. Some
artists sketch it out in the rough. They begin to paint accepting any happy accidents or organic changes as they come. I often begin with a very
simple design rendering that is complemented by a vision in my mind. I

paint in little pieces. It is almost like one of those invisible magic drawing books. My Aunts placed those books in my Christmas stocking as a child. I would rub a quarter or a pencil over nothing and then parts of an elaborate drawing would appear. What magic! There was a drawing all along and I just could not see it. The composition of a life is like that. We rarely get to see the big picture when we are living it. Life doesn't always work out like we plan and we finish parts of the picture at different times. In 2008, I was living in the rough sketch, completely unaware that the big picture would soon be revealed

I watched *Doctor Who* a lot as a youngster. I watched every episode of the Tom Baker and Peter Davidson years on my local PBS station. In sixth grade, I created a piece of art in which my first name forms the image of a space alien. Surrounding the alien is the Doctor with his TARDIS, a poster from the mini-series *V,* and a hospital standing high in the sky with ambulance ships flying in. A shuttle with a sign that says "Just Married" flies by. I drew this in 1986. As the Doctor would say, time is in flux. Some things can be changed and some are fixed points. It is hard to see God's plan when you are living it. Just like River Song said in "Forest of the Dead," everything was leading to this time, to this moment.

When I became an adult, time passed quickly and life grew busy. I fell out of touch with *Doctor Who.* In 2005 my loving husband Fred, told me it was making a comeback on the BBC. I think I said, "Oh, that's nice." I was too busy with work and child care to worry about a fictional character on television. With Isaac born in 2006, I had absolutely no free time. A new fellow named Will Kemp was hired while I was on my maternity four weeks at the toy store. Upon my return, he was always making comments about the Doctor. I would listen politely, and then go on to more important things.

In July of 2008, I was home alone. When Fred and the boys were in the house it was so noisy. They ran and played. Fred would either watch *The West Wing, Scrubs* or *The Daily Show* in a fairly constant rotation. When Fred and the boys would leave for a weekend to visit grandpa Fred and grandma Joan, I would silence the TV and read in my scant spare time. For some reason, during this time of solitude I instead turned to the Sci-Fi channel and saw the second part in a two-part episode of *Doctor Who.* This wasn't just any old episode. I had grown up watching the Doctor. I knew the mythos. No one knows the Doctor's name, No one. Who was this woman? Was this woman the Doctor's wife? I sat in rapt attention as the drama unfolded. Tears ran down my face as I watched her die. I was so touched and inspired.

I called Fred. I was talking a mile a minute. I described the show and asked him questions. We agreed we would watch the entire series starting with the episodes from 2005. Fred chuckled at my happiness and said, "Reggie, I haven't heard you this excited in years." Fred, Freddie and Isaac came home, and we began our journey to the new world of Doctor Who. Each night we would watch an episode to try to catch up. It was so much fun. Fred and I were really enjoying watching the series. Our joy spread to the children. They began to watch and play-act Doctor Who. It wasn't long before Freddie decided that this show would be his birthday party theme. We agreed our family Halloween costumes would be Who-inspired as well.

Our friendships were affected by this new interest. I got to know Will from work much better as we had numerous conversations about the Doctor. He told me different ways to research the show online. I had never ventured out much on the internet; but with this new interest, I learned much more about Wiki's and Youtube and Google alerts. After Fred started his fall semester at AU, we went to a faculty party. There we mentioned our fan status. Fred didn't know many people at the party. When we mentioned *Doctor Who,* we were introduced to Michael and Rebecca. Michael Wenthe worked in the Literature Dept. at American University and Rebecca Boggs was his wife. They were great fans of *Doctor Who.* I mentioned we wanted to have a Doctor Who themed birthday party for our eldest. Would they be interested in helping? Sure, they said. I could Facebook message them the details. I walked away a bit worried because I did not know how to Facebook.

Planning the *Doctor Who* party forced me to become familiar with Facebook. I found it be a great resource for coordination of such a large undertaking. There would be 70 children at the party, half of them special education students. I would need many adults to help supervise activities. I also got in touch with people I had known through the years. These were people I thought had the skill set to help with such a complicated party. We had been out of touch, but through Facebook became close again. The party was amazing, and it was a magical night. It all came together so well. This was a party for a Time Lord, and anyone in time or space was invited. The children and adults had a ball dressing as their favorite characters. So many wonderful people came to celebrate. Our interest in the show continued into the rest of the fall and winter.

For Halloween 2008 we donned costumes once again. I was a Dalek. I designed my costume so a Razor scooter could fit underneath. If you happened to be on Connecticut Avenue on October 31, 2008, you would have seen a Dalek rolling by. Freddie was the Tenth Doctor complete with sonic screwdriver, and Isaac was Captain Jack Harkness riding a "Face of Boe" Kettler push-style tricycle. Fred was our cameraman. I think about four people recognized our costumes, but we were so happy.

After Halloween, we were still interested in the show. Freddie wanted to make Doctor Who action figure movies. Fred and I agreed to take our Christmas money and get a family video camera. So at Christmas 2008 we filmed the boys opening their Doctor Who gifts, with Fred's running commentary in the background. We also heard that David Tennant would not be playing the Doctor after 2009. There would be five specials in 2009 with Tenant; then he would regenerate. Fred and I bemoaned the fact we became obsessed with the show in a year with so few episodes. How would we make it through 2009?

That seems so long ago.

So Much Pain

THE FALL OF 2008 WAS filled with our new joy in *Doctor Who* and Fred's increasing physical pain. Throughout the fall Fred was fatigued and he ached. He decided to go to the doctor. Fred had been uninsured for many years and he went to a doctor's office that had been a clinic that accepted the uninsured. When he finally got insurance he decided to continue being treated at this office. When he went in that fall he was diagnosed with hypertension. I thought that diagnosis very odd as throughout the summer Fred was dropping weight. He liked his new slim look so much he began to exercise and eat very healthy choices to continue the weight loss. I wondered why he would have hypertension now when he was so close to his ideal weight.

During that fall, I was new to Facebook. I enjoyed posting simple status lines and responding to my husband. I did not like Facebook games and would not play them. Fred loved them, and I am glad he did. Through the list memes of 2009 he can speak to all of us still today:

"A-z pass along" by Frederick Holliday, Wednesday, February 4, 2009 at 10:20pm

"Sorry to you all, but I just can't help myself (though I was able to refrain from tagging my dear wife who has made it quite clear she does NOT like these note-memes). This one is pretty self-explanatory. If you do it, have fun. If you don't, how can I stop? Please God I wanna stop!

A

- Available: nope
- Age: 38 (for a little less than two more months)
- Annoyance: Mostly myself
- Animal: dogs
- Actor: Right now, Bruno Ganz

B

- Beer: A fond memory from my past
- Birthday/Birthplace: March 31, 1970, Cumberland MD
- Best Friends: (historically) Alex Hicks, Greg Holtschneider (though the creep refuses to facebook), Jeff Miller, Chris Meissner
- Body Part on desired sex: brain
- Best feeling in the world: Isaac and Freddie laughing together
- Best weather: Warm spring Saturday
- Been in Love: Still am
- Been on stage?: yes, I was a theatre major once upon a time.
- Believe in yourself?: yes and no. mostly no.
- Believe in life on other planets: Of course.
- Believe in miracles: define the term more specifically and I'll answer. I've seen some darn strange things, but they just as easily could have been coincidences.
- Believe in magic: no
- Believe in God: yes, but I've got a lot of questions for him/her
- Believe in Satan: yes
- Believe in Santa: no
- Believe in ghosts/spirits: See my answer to the "miracles" question.
- Believe in evolution: without a damn doubt!

C

- Car: 2004 Chevy Cava-something, I don't know cars. We're buying a new one soon.
- Candy: Twix
- Color: oddly enough, olive green
- Cried in school: Ahahahahahahahaha (that's for all my undergrad friends out there!)
- Chinese/Mexican: wo fei chang xi.huan zhong.guo fan.le!
- Cake or pie: pumpkin pie is the most delicious thing on the whole damn planet! (Apologies to Donkey)
- Country to visit: Britain or China

D

- Day or Night: Night better TV
- Dream vehicle: don't really have one
- Dance: not if my life depended on it
- Dance in the rain?: nope
- Do the splits?: are you kidding?

E

- Eggs: Over easy, scrambled, or hard-boiled.
- Eyes: Blue
- Ever failed a class? A few. Most esp. high school geometry where I actually competed to get the lowest grade in the course.
- First crush: Andrea Nofziger (age 2 6)
- Full name: Frederick Allen Holliday II
- First thoughts waking up: Are the boys up yet?
- Food: meat, glorious meat.

G

- Greatest Fear: something happening to my boys
- Giver or taker: No comment
- Goals: Find more permanent full time work
- Gum: very very rarely

- Get along with your parents?: very much!
- Good luck charm: Russian bill given to me by the great John Carter Tibbetts!
- The perfect Guy: Weirdly, David Mamet

H

- Hair: all but gone... dammit!
- Height: 5'8"
- Happy: varies
- Holiday: Christmas, though the reason has shifted in the last decade
- How do you want to die: while sleeping
- Health freak?: Not as much as I'd like, though better than I used to be.
- Hate: the inability to value an opinion different from one's own.

I

- Ice Cream: cookies'n'cream
- Instrument: none

J

- Jewelry: Wedding Ring
- Job: Best one in the world!

K

- Kids: 2 great boys!
- Kickboxing or karate: neither
- Keep a journal?: no, my memory's currently pretty good.

L

- Love: Reg, Reg, Reg. She's taught me all I know about it.
- Letter: F (it has so many uses)
- Laughed so hard you cried: Issac: "I not nice. I ANGRY!!!!!!!!"
- Love at first sight: Actually, yeah. It's how I fell for Regina.

M

- Milk flavor: I no longer drink milk
- Movie: Changes from minute-to-minute
- Mooned anyone?: Good God no. That wouldn't be good for anyone!
- Marriage: 15 years last 12/26
- Motion sickness? no
- McD's or BK: FIVE FRIGGIN' GUYS

N

- Number of siblings: two, though we barely speak.
- Number of piercings: none
- Number: 24fps

O

- Overused phrases: Know what I mean?
- One wish: happiness for my boys
- Phobia: Too many to list (highlights: heights, tornados, social situations, small spaces)

P

- Place you'd like to live: NYC for a little while anyway
- Perfect Pizza: Armands
- Pepsi/Coke: I no longer drink soda

Q

- Quail: Yummy, but a rare meal for me.
- Questionnaires: Revealing and fun. Also: annoying.

R

- Reason to cry: Oh I don't know.. maybe a friggin' broken rib!
- Reality TV: I'd rather take a melon-baller to my eyes!
- Radio Station: WAMU
- Roll your tongue in a circle? Yes.

S
- Song: New Years Day and Don't Change
- Shoe size: 9 1/2
- Salad Dressing: dry please
- Sushi: yuck
- Skipped school: Oh my yes. My undergrad GPA is shameful as a result
- Slept outside: only when I have to
- Seen a dead body? Yes
- Smoked?: Nope
- Skinny dipped?: Nope
- Shower daily?: Yes
- Sing well? Oh no. No no no.
- Stuffed Animals?: When I was a kid I had an entire rep company.
- Single/Group dates: Both
- Strawberries/Blueberries: Strawberries, but no damn sugar thank you.

T
- Time for bed: varies, but usually 12 or 1
- Thunderstorms: hate them with the white hot fury of fear
- TV Show: Battlestar Galactica
- Touch your tongue to your nose: Not even close

U
- Unpredictable: you never know.

V
- Vegetable you hate: pickles
- Vegetable you love: lima beans (Yeah, I said it!)
- Vacation spot: For the last 8 years or so, Enid Oklahoma -the second coolest non-east coast place in the US!

W

- Weakness: disorganization
- When you grow up: When will that finally happen? For the love of God when?
- Which one of your friends acts the most like you: Thankfully, none. They're all better than me.
- Who makes you laugh the most: Isaac
- Worst feeling: fear. it rules me.
- Wanted to be a model?: Yeah. the "Before" guy.
- Worst weather: Tornado season

X

- X-Rays: Inconclusive. Dammit!

Y

- Year it is now: 2009
- Yellow: A great episode of TALES FROM THE CRYPT directed by Robert Zemekis (SP?)

Z

- Zoo animal: Panda (Go DC!)
- Zodiac sign: Aries... whatever the hell that means."

I laughed at Fred's funny posts. I responded to all his queries. But I did not scroll down pages of his content to see a pattern of disease. If I had data-mined my husband's posts in 2008 through 2009, I would have seen so many symptoms of disease; but we were living in the rough sketch and I did not see the larger picture.

In January of 2009, the entire family had a very bad cold. All of us were coughing on a daily basis. Soon Fred's ribs hurt so badly he went to the ER. The staff at the ER said he had broken them coughing. I thought it unusual that he had broken ribs by just coughing. This was an irritating cough, but not an explosive one. I went to my doctor with the same cough and got antibiotics. I told my primary about Fred's broken ribs as he listened to my lungs. The doctor asked how old was Fred. I told my doctor Fred was 38 years old. My doctor's brows furrowed as he said, "If it were one of my geriatric patients, I would not be too alarmed, but in a 38 year old male I would look for an underlying problem." Fred brought up my concerns with his doctor, but Fred's doctor brushed off my worries and prescribed pain medication.

By February 2009, Fred had a new complaint; he was suffering from excruciating lower back pain. The doctor thought he might be suffering from a protuberance of lumbar five. She gave him more pain meds, but she forgot to prescribe laxative. So now we had a new problem. While I was in Navy boot camp in the summer of 1993, I remembered I had heard a very important lecture. It was a week and a half into Boot camp and the CPO (Chief Petty Officer) wanted to talk to us girls about our bowels. We sat in silence. She said, "I know a lot of you have changed your diet and are frightened. You may not have had many bowel movements or have had none. This is dangerous. If you do not have a bowel movement you will become impacted and could end up needing surgery. If you have not had a bowel movement in several days, please report to the doctor." I was so glad she spoke to us. I had not had a bowel movement in two weeks. I was embarrassed and did not know what to do.

Fred was taking a great deal of pain medication and became very constipated. He was embarrassed. I told him about my boot camp experience and urged him to go back to the doctor about the constipation. By the time he went back to the doctor, he was more concerned about the constipation than the back pain. She gave him a laxative, then more pain medication and then more laxatives. By March 2009, Fred was on four types of pain medications, two muscle relaxants and four laxatives. We had no confirmed diagnosis of what was causing Fred so much pain.

When we were not dealing with pain that spring, we were dealing with an excessive amount of art. It was school auction time and I was working with a multitude of schools. Most years Fred would cut out hundreds of children's art pieces to help me create gigantic collage canvases that held a class creation. This spring Fred was mostly lying down when at home. It hurt a great deal to sit up, so he could do very little cutting. He would talk with me while I cut painted flowers and that was nice. Our very small apartment was filled with canvases as the auction days drew near. Fred and I attended the CCBC auction, and he looked very nice in his suit, but oh, so very tired. As the evening of our annual date progressed, Fred told me he hurt so very much. We left early and Fred would lie down the moment we returned home.

March 13, 2009 was a Friday. Fred came home from work in so much pain that he was crying. I told Fred, "Let's go to the ER. They will have to find out what is wrong with you." We packed a bag of toys and little plastic dinosaurs and we took the boys with us. We went to the hospital with the pretty ER. There were lovely blue couches, stained glass windows, a gift shop and a coffee shop. We sat and waited for three hours while the children played. Finally someone came out from express wound care. They explained that the testing rooms were overloaded with patients. We would get no MRI or CAT scan. They told us they were concerned that Fred might be anemic and recommended we see Fred's regular doctor the next week. They also gave us more pain meds.

The next week I went with Fred to the doctor.

I always acted as an advocate for my children at the doctor's office. I would ask questions and make sure I understood treatment protocols. I never thought I would have to do that for my husband, but after six months of watching Fred deteriorate little by little, I decided I must go with him to the appointment. Fred did not like to make waves or question authority, so he was very stressed out that I would antagonize his doctor by asking too many questions. When we arrived to what was an almost weekly appointment, the nurse just told us to enter the examination room. I asked, "Aren't you going to weigh him?" As someone who has spent most of my life overweight, I know my doctors always weighed me and would follow up with a conversation about my weight. The nurse responded that they do not always weigh their patients. I turned around and said, "Well, then how do you know he is losing weight? He is losing weight. I know because I am his wife and see him naked. You need to weigh your patients to track their weight gain or loss. This can be a sign of disease."

She just ushered us into the room. Fred rested upon the exam table while we waited for the doctor. A few moments later the doctor entered the room, her eyes downcast as she was reading Fred's paper chart. She flipped paper over paper as she asked Fred, "So do you think that maybe you're depressed?" Fred looked at her with an incredulous face. I responded indignantly, "Of course he is depressed! He is in excruciating pain and has been for months. I think there is something wrong with his kidneys."

The doctor looked at me her eyebrow arched as she said, "I am pretty sure this pain is the result of a protruding lumbar five. Some people are not bothered by it and some need surgery." I responded. "We want an MRI. Fred has come to you for months and you have no confirmed diagnosis for his pain. We want an MRI this week and it needs to be something called an open MRI. Fred is claustrophobic." I could not understand why she had not ordered an MRI sooner. Had she forgotten Fred was insured and was concerned we could not pay for it? The doctor left the room to find a list of local MRI clinics that could see Fred that week.

There was an open MRI in Olney, Maryland, that could see Fred. He drove all the way out of DC to the bedroom community of Olney. They did a scan of Fred's lower back as requested by his primary care physician. The Olney staff created a CD of his imaging results for Fred to give to his doctor. Fred drove towards home and dropped the CD off at his doctor's office on the way. She called us four days later.

Life In A Box

ON TUESDAY MARCH 24, I was at church with Isaac. Fred had left to teach class and Freddie was in school. It must have been spring break at CCBC. Isaac was "helping" me clean up a storage area at church in preparation for our rummage sale in May. We had recently begun having a rummage sale each spring and fall at St. Paul's Lutheran Church in Washington, DC.

In the fall of 2008, I prepared for my first rummage sale to help the homeless shelter at St. Paul's Lutheran Church. As the piles of donated goods slowly filled the portico off sanctuary, a space that was usually empty, still, and sacred became filled with bric-a-brac. These were the "extra things," the things easily given away to help those who had lost all they had. As I sorted and priced item after item, a lovely woman with an assured stance, strode into the room with a box. "I no longer need these," she said. I gave her a tax receipt and laid the box aside. Later that evening, I began to sort through the box. It was mostly books. In the box was a newlywed's guide to cooking for two, a book on how to please your man and an adult board game bought from Spencer's Gifts. I chuckled a bit at the game and priced it at a dollar, as ELCA Lutherans are a pretty accepting bunch.

Then I pulled out more books: a hardback book about how to know if he is cheating, a guide to navigate divorce, a dog-eared paperback on grief. The chuckle died upon my lips. Finally, I lifted out a book about positive thinking and a hardback about being a single empowered woman.

I smiled at the final titles, and looked down at all that had been given. This was a life in a box. Life is filled with transitions such as the ones represented by this donation. Some times such transitions span years and decades. Sometimes they span only weeks. In hospital settings I would learn that such transitions often end the same way, with a life in a box.

After a long morning of cleaning, Isaac and I headed home for an early lunch. I was spreading peanut butter and jelly on Wonder bread when Fred stumbled through the door partially supported by his friend and fellow colleague, Michael Wenthe. Michael helped Fred to the couch. Fred had tried to teach class that day. At American University the teacher's parking lot is quite far from the classroom space. At this point Fred's pain was intolerable even with the medications he was taking. Fred made it halfway across the lot, before he had to lower himself to the pavement. Michael had found him on the ground. He called the University and told them Fred was sick, and he drove Fred home in our car. As Michael and Fred explained this all to me, the phone rang. It was Fred's doctor. Her voice was curt. She said that she had looked at the CD and wanted us to make an appointment with an oncologist she knew the next day. She told me his number, and then click she hung up the phone. I wasn't even sure what an oncologist was. I looked that up online. It is a cancer doctor.

We called Fred's mother Joan to come to DC and made an appointment to see the doctor early the next morning on March 25. Fred drove the car even though he was hurting so much, as I did not drive. Our appointment was in the physician's building attached to the hospital that had the pretty ER we had visited less than two weeks before. Fred winced with pain as he walked to the doctor's office. We had the first appointment of the day and the receptionist waved us in. Fred gasped a bit as he tried to sit on the examination table.

The doctor came in. He told us he had looked at the CD containing the MRI of Fred's lower back. Fred's doctor had requested an image of the region around lumbar five. The lower parts of Fred's kidneys were visible in the image. The oncologist was concerned because he could see a shadow on the kidneys. He wanted to order an MRI and CAT scan of Fred's lower abdomen. The doctor explained to Fred that he should be admitted, because that would expedite the tests. We waited in the lobby for hours until they found a bed for Fred. They finally got him in a room and the nurses asked about which medications Fred was taking. I admitted that he was taking so many that I was not sure of their names and types. She told me I would have to go home and get them.

That was far easier said then done. I left the hospital and walked several blocks to the nearest Metro station. I then took the metro from Maryland looping around downtown DC and all the way to the Van Ness/ Chevy Chase neighborhood where we lived. I rushed upstairs and gathered all of Fred's many pills. I picked up Freddie from school. Then Joan, Freddie, Isaac and I took the bus, then the Metro and finally walk up the hill to Fred's bed in the hospital. I gave the nurse a bag containing bottles of medication. I brought from home 26 tablets of Hydrocodone-apap 5-500 (a substitute for Vicodin), Skelaxin 800mg 11 ½ tablets, Cyclobenzaprine 10 mg 5 tablets, Naproxen Sodium 550 mg, 5 tablets, Atacand HCT 32-12.5mg 9 tablets, Ultram ER (tramadol HCI) 100mg 18 tablets (an opioid not recommended in cases of renal impairment, and should not be used with severe renal impairment), AcipHex-rabeprazole sodium 20mg 21 tablets, Senna 8.6mg 38 tablets left from a jar of 100, and Miralax 17g 2 of 14 doses left. She did not record the laxatives. Fred had regular movements again prior to going to the hospital. When the nurse took his medication history she was only interested in the prescription drugs. She said they would handle laxatives if they were needed. Fred had been stable on the four laxatives. They stopped them all.

After the nurse recorded the types of prescription medicine brought from home, these were left in the room with Fred. They were not locked in a secure location, as is the case at most hospitals. I placed them in the closet, as I was not sure where they needed to go. In the days after diagnosis, I would worry a great deal about those pills in a room with Fred. Fred's admission screening did not include my husband's history of depression. After Fred received his upsetting diagnosis, no additional crises intervention was offered. When he mentioned suicidal thoughts to me in the coming weeks, I thought it prudent to remove the medications from his room.

We stayed with Fred a few more hours on that Wednesday to keep up his spirits. Then Joan drove the boys and me home in the family car. She parked it near the apartment building on a side street and there it would sit for the next two months. I would visit Fred during the each day and we would all bemoan how long it was taking to complete the tests. We would nervously chat and bring Fred lots of chocolate pudding from the cafeteria.

I was working a shift at the toy store on Friday, March 27. I was help ing a family pick out a birthday gift in the art department. Fred was at the hospital getting tests to determine the cause of his back pain. He was just getting tests. I did not know that you should not leave patients alone in a hospital. Then Fred called. My husband called so many times in the twelve years I had worked at Child's Play. It was almost a running joke. How many times would Fred call today? I refused to own a cell phone, so Fred's calling would tie up our main phone line at work. My boss, Steven, would often hand me the phone with a look of massive frustration and say, "It's Fred. Again." This time there was no frustration, only concern, as the phone was handed to me.

Can a phone become a snake? Can it bite and strike? I think it can. As a child, I loved the curling spiral of the cord. I would wrap my fingers within its nestled coils and wonder. As a teen, I would spin round and round while speaking to my boyfriend at the other end of the line. As I spun in circles, slowly the cord would wrap me in a constricting embrace. But the toy store phone was cordless and dark. It was a regular phone. I answered it, and I cried.

Fred sounded so worried. He was crying as he told me, "The Doctor says I have tumors and growths in my abdomen and a 3cm tumor in my kidney. Please come as soon as you can, Reggie. I am so scared." His words rang within my mind. His voice was choked with emotion as we said goodbye. I asked my coworker Simmie to drive me to the hospital as I did not drive and needed to get there quickly. Most of Simmie's family worked in medicine, and as she drove she gave advice. She told me to write everything down that was happening when I got to the hospital. She said I would need to be Fred's record keeper. When we arrived, I thanked her and rushed to Fred's side. I hugged him and tried to learn more about what the doctor had said. Fred was very upset and could recall few details. I went to the nurses' station and asked to see Fred's doctor. The nurse told me the doctor had left for a medical conference and would be gone for the next four days. He would not reply to my emails or calls while at the conference. The nurse told me Fred was scheduled to have more tests. He was scheduled for a PET scan and a bone scan that weekend. After the results came in they would know about spread. Until then we would wait.

Waiting

WHEN I WAS A LITTLE girl, I would stare for hours at the wooden clock upon the wall at my Aunt Minnie's house. I found it quite intriguing. The clock was a little house with a bird that would dip its beak outside its window and cuckoo upon the hour. A little wooden boy and a little wooden girl would meet in front of their doors, share a kiss, then depart. The clock seemed magical and full of hope. The sun would always rise, the bird would always tweet, and the girl and boy would always kiss. But life is not like woodwork clocks with metal pinecone counterweights. Life is unpredictable and sometimes you wake up to find the timepiece is still ticking but the boy is lost forever. Some people think we live in linear time. Those of us who have spent time in hospitals know better. We know that the weeks turn into days, and the caregiving continues even as the mind tries to escape.

The weekend of March 28-29, we found friends willing to watch the children. My father-in-law, Fred and mother-in-law, Joan waited with Fred and me to hear the test results. We waited with Fred in his room when he was awake, but as he slept we would go to the cafeteria or the waiting room down the hall. The 6th floor oncology waiting room was a dark depressing place. The overhead light was usually turned off and the visitors would wait in darkness. The waiting room was adjacent to a busy hallway with an elevator. Bells and buzzers could be heard down the hall, each chirping a warning before the nurse pressed the silence button. Mixed with the clamor of bells and buzzers was the odor of ammonia and incontinence. The housekeepers would wage war upon this embarrassing odor with an arsenal of antiseptic sprays and bleach. The toxic specks of sprayed cleaners danced with the dust motes in the air, creating a nauseating cloud.

The room was devoid of any form of entertainment or distraction from grief. There was no remote for the forlorn TV that rested upon a low shelf. It was stuck displaying the endless hell of C-SPAN. The button that changed the channel was gone, leaving a gaping hole in the base of the set. When I asked a nurse how did one change the channels, she recommended sticking a ballpoint pen in the gaping hole. As the pen had a metal casing, I decided to forgo her advice. The TV could be made louder or quieter, but it could not change. It could only be turned off. The reading material consisted of a few glossy corporate magazines provided by pharmaceutical companies. In these periodicals, breast cancer patients got 25 pages devoted to their disease; kidney cancer got a paragraph.

An elderly nun often sat in the darkened corner dressed in a volunteer's smock. Snoring gently, she slumped back with her mouth open. An errant line of spittle flew back and forth between her lips. Other visitors whispered quietly into their cell phones. Occasionally their voices would break and become audible. A staff person trudged into the room and sat alone at the long table. She pulled food containers out of a disposable blue grocery bag. She stared into space and shoveled the food into her mouth. The people in this room were separate and alone. No one made eye contact. This waiting room existed to provide a space to give up fragile hope and choice. This was a place where plans and life paths were destroyed and every element combined to create a despairing world of erasure.

Joan and I would happily leave that dismal waiting room and return to Fred. There we would wait at his side until the on call doctor finally visited the room. She walked in the room barely greeting us she went over to check Fred's PCA pump. She was confirming the bolus amount as we stared at her and finally asked, "What about the test results? Fred had a PET scan and a bone scan and we have been waiting to hear the results." She looked at each of us in turn and said, "You mean no one has told you? The cancer has spread. It is everywhere. It is in his lungs and bones."

That night I went home to my computer and realized he was at stage 4 of kidney cancer. The median survival rate at his stage of disease was 12 weeks to six months.

The Final Paper

My husband, Fred, was so proud to get his dream job. He had gone to school for many years to achieve a Doctorate of Film Studies. He loved working at American University in his one year appointed position split between the Department of the Performing Arts and the Department of Literature. He was so happy. With deep regret Fred realized he could no longer teach and would need to hand off his classes to another teacher. I offered to help put his class papers in order. In the next two days I learned that Fred was a great teacher. A life can be defined by the work that we do and it is important to show up and do a good job.

The first task Fred assigned me was to clean out his desk in the office he shared with another professor. When Fred was hired he was told that he would share an office with a department head in the performing arts department. Fred was aghast that he would be invading her personal space. He was always gracious to her and kept his time in the office to just required office hours. He tried not to clutter up her space with any of his personal things. He placed no pictures on his desk, and no mementos reminded her of his presence. I went over to American on a quiet Saturday. No one was in the building. I let myself in the door to his office. I had brought two bags with me. It did not take long to fill them with all the papers and attendance sheets for his performing arts classes. I closed the drawers and looked at his empty desk and cried.

I did not have to clean out his desk in the Literature Department. They had no office space for him. He had used the department lounge for his office hours. There he had wonderful conversations with students and other faculty members, but there was no space to break down. There was only the memory of him sitting there and laughing and talking about film. I completed the first task with a sense of longing and remorse; my eyes scanned the halls and said goodbye.

Fred assigned a second task; I was to gather up all the papers and emails from home. This was a far more complex task. Fred's desk was a pile of papers. It was his tiny kingdom in our very small apartment. I was not supposed to touch his papers or straighten them. His filing system may have looked a mess but he had it organized in his own special way. The time had come to violate his space and shut down his home office. I shuffled all of these piles of papers together and placed them in new bags. Fred also had messenger bags full of papers separated by class and department under the desk. I gathered them up. I called him at the hospital and asked him, "Is there anything else? " "Yes," he said. "You need to log on to my email and print out any late papers submitted through Blackboard." I also printed out any emails explaining past absences. While searching for these missives, I read an email from a past student asking for a letter of recommendation. I called Fred again. He had already written the letter and told me how to find the file to print it out. I placed all of these copies in the bags of office detritus. I gathered the remnants of a life's work and rolled them out of our living room in my shopping pushcart. I had completed task two; and left behind me a gaping wound masquerading as a clean desk in our living room.

Fred and I worked for hours on the last task of preparing all his papers and attendance records in order to hand over his class to two other teachers. I stood beside him using the hospital tray as a desk. He would call out names from attendance sheets and I would make the tally mark. He told me after six absences the student's grade would be affected. As I watched the tally marks grow, I began to root for certain students. I kept hoping I would not hear their name again. Time wore on and certain names had seven or eight absences marked. I became mad at those students. How dare they skip class? Why did they miss this opportunity to learn from this great teacher? He was slowly dying of cancer, and he had come to class. What excuse could they have for seven absences? Finally we finished the tally.

It was time to grade the late papers. Fred graded slowly and deliberately. When he got to the last paper, he turned his face to me. He said, "Reg, this is too well written for this student. Please take it to one of the hospital computers and type a line into Google." I took the paper down the hall. I typed the first line into the Google search field. The hospital's ethical mission statement barred me from the original site of the paper, but I could see it was a plagiarized paper. I went back and told Fred. He marked that fact on the paper and we placed it in the neat pile of papers that represented lives.

We had finished the job of a teacher. The piles of work awaited the new instructor. We sat in the twilight holding hands, proud of our accomplishment. Fred would live for 11 more weeks, but his life's work ended that day. This was the last day he did his job. He was proud and sad. He loved his students and missed them. I looked over at him with great love and respect. He had come to class even as he was dying. He agonized over his students' attendance and tried to show them how to do their best. He showed us all in his final days how important it is to do your work and to remember not to get marked absent in the class of life.

The Kingdom Of The Sick

WHEN I WAS YOUNG, I had a compulsion to find out how things worked. This usually led to creative destruction. I know exactly how a music box works because I dismantled my jewelry box, tossing out the painted pasteboard, the velveteen lining and the plastic ballerina. The important part was inside. I loved the little brass machine that wound with a key. I loved to listen to the metallic plinks as the metal keys were forced upon the raised nodules of the rotating barrel. I cherished the simple elegance hidden for years by the bulky form of the jewelry box. It was liberating.

But my deconstruction did not stop with the music box. I also wanted to see inside a mirror. Mirrors were amazing things that created a world in reverse. One day I ripped the brown paper backing off of my mirror. Then I scraped at the black paint on the back of the glass. My scraping revealed a silver expanse. I scraped at that layer and reached clear transparent glass. I was disappointed. I could not see inside the mirror. I could not see that most amazing space between the darkness and the glass. I knew that was where the magic happened. I knew another world lived inside the glass.

I want you to think about how many times a day you look within a mirror. Every time we enter a bathroom we glance in the mirror to double check our appearance. We use mirrors to take those lovely photos that create avatars on countless social media sites. We stride upon the streets of a city, and reflected upon endless windowpanes a dark copy of our face walks beside us marking time.

Someone once asked me how to show regular people what it feels like to be a bedridden patient. I responded, "That is easy. Cover every hall and bathroom mirror with black paper." The person asking for my advice looked at me quizzically and waited for my explanation. "The very compromised patient is stuck in his or her bed. Most hospital bedside tray tables do not have a mirror, or if they do it is often broken. So you spend a lot of time alone without even the comforting gaze of your own eyes."

Hospitals can deconstruct a person as assuredly as I could lay bare a jewelry box. Take any professional adult and remove their clothes and their accessories. Dress them in a threadbare gown that is faded by thousands of wash cycles. Give them a number rather than a name. Confuse them with jargon whist applying copious amounts medication. Then watch them try to navigate the maze of care.

Hospitals are very hard to navigate when well, let alone sick, and the learning curve of a patient and family caregiver is a steep and painful one. Fred and I thought we were on the oncology floor because ONCOLOGY was written on the wall in large letters right across from the elevator, but we were in a general admissions room. We were confused at our nurses seeming inability to understand the multiple problems my husband was facing. We found out we were on the "*wrong*" side of the hallway on April 9. The oncologist decided to move us to the oncology side of the hall, as Fred would be starting radiation treatment soon. Finally, oncology-trained nurses would treat him. We had been in the hospital for 16 days at this point with Metastatic Renal Cell Carcinoma.

On March 27, 2009 when we found out Fred's body had tumors and growths, I still had several art auction pieces I needed to finish. The night of the 27th I finished the piece for the Little Flowers School. It was a Warhol inspired self-portrait series of the entire kindergarten class. The Auction was the next day. There was no more time to waste. I heard later that that piece went for several hundred dollars. I wonder if the owners have any idea how valuable it really is? Normally, when I adhere rice paper onto canvas I use a lot of water and gel medium. This time I used gel medium and tears. I cried for all of our lost tomorrows on that bright canvas.

As the days passed by Fred grew worse and could barely get out of bed. My husband tried to support all his weight on a rolling IV tower at his nurse's suggestion. (This advice does not reflect the fall prevention guidelines at most hospitals.) He was encouraged to go to the bathroom by himself even when the marble lip that joined the floor of the bathroom to the patient room required wrangling of the IV tower over the bump. I had trouble completing this feat with no disability. As my husband lost the ability to walk this became impossible. He lay in his hospital bed. My husband stopped walking on 4-08-09. We did not understand it at the time, but when he could no longer walk surgery was no longer an option. No one from physical therapy would come help Fred, no ortho consult was provided to help with ambulation. If we had been able to read the medical record, we would have seen "ortho is forthcoming," but they never came. The medical record also specified a request for a walker. The walker was never provided.

I sat beside Fred and began to cut out the cherry blossoms that Mrs. Schaffer's 2nd grade class at Murch Elementary had painted onto rice paper. These were part of a composition that framed an acrylic painting of the Washington Monument in cherry branches. It had been a cool spring. Outside the cherry blossoms were just beginning to unfold. Fred looked over at me. My lap was filled with painted paper flowers. "I guess I will miss seeing the cherry blossoms this year," he said. I looked up at him. He continued, "I hope I am here to seem them next year." I looked down quickly and continued cutting so Fred would not see my eyes fill with tears. The next day I brought the finished painting to Mrs. Schaffer's Class. The teachers circled around me and held me close as I sobbed. Other than the few glimpses of flowers Fred saw during his ambulance transports for radiation, Fred would never see cherry blossoms again.

When Fred was in the hospital, I was always writing in a journal. I noted the procedures that were happening and noted who came in the room. I also would sketch simple pictures and write poetry. I thought about a fellow parent who had recently died of cancer. Her name was Elika Hemphill. I helped her at the toy store for many years. I was so excited to see her become an involved parent at my son's school. I watched her fight her first round of cancer while taking care of a family. When she went into remission she came by the store one day and asked me to paint a mural of her children's faces on her fence just like my mural work at American City Diner. I said I would as soon as my schedule freed up. My schedule did not free up in time for Elika to get her painting. She came in the toy store on June 25, 2008. She was in a hurry, but I asked her if she would like to enroll her children in the art lesson I was teaching the next day. She said yes. She came even though she had received devastating news. Her cancer was back. She would die in the fall of 2008. I wrote this poem about her as I watched my husband sleep.

The Last Time I saw Elika

The last time I saw Elika,
Sunlight-Shining Elika,
She sat on the bench and looked away
And as she sat her children played.
They painted cherry blossom scenes
And she looked upon them in between.

The day I heard, oh Elika,
Michelle told me, oh Elika
The cancer's back and now has spread.
It's gone through her. It's in her head.
Oh no...Oh why? This isn't fair!
But these thoughts, I did not share.

Why not go see Elika?
I could not go see Elika.
I could not bear to think
Her face not now so rosy pink.
Her sunlight-shine begun to fade.
And all the hope is now forbade.

Each time I thought of her I cried
Like some part inside of me had died.
Maybe my heart already knew,
My crying time was coming soon.
That my sunlight-shining day would end.
That I would lose my greatest friend.

She knew she'd die that painting day.
She knew, and she came anyway.
Because it's worth it one last time
To see the sun, to paint, to shine,
To be with children and to show
How much you love them as you go.

-Regina Holliday 4-7-09

The Little Things

My mother hated her initials the entire time she worked as a hospital housekeeper. Her initials are "BM." Ha, ha that is a great joke in a hospital. She hated to write those initials and know that others were smirking. She was deeply embarrassed by the coincidence of letters. They represented her identity and represented the messes she cleaned off the floor. It was not a joke to her.

Have you ever potty trained a child or a puppy? It can be a long and drawn out process. You might have a sticker chart or prizes for every time your little one succeeds. You might use shame for every time they do not. I never understood that phrase "rubbing your nose in it" until I saw a friend potty train her dog. The shame of incontinence is instilled at a very young age. And the shame does not stop there. Children grow up aware of society's aversion to talking about bowel problems or urinary mistakes.

The entry about incontinence from Wikipedia stated, "Fecal incontinence is the loss of regular control of the bowels. Involuntary excretion and leaking are common occurrences for those affected. Subjects relating to defecation are often socially unacceptable, thus those affected may be beset by feelings of shame and humiliation." My Fred indeed suffered "shame and humiliation" with this new condition. I would even say he worried more about this element of his condition that he worried about the cancer itself. No therapist ever comes to your side to talk about this shame. No one explains the process of why this is happening to your body. No one wants to talk about it.

When I was with Fred I did his bedding changes when he had a movement. When I was not there, I had to depend on medical technicians and nurses to do this duty. I would sometimes arrive and find him sitting in filth. In one case a nurse had just been in the room. I asked her why hadn't she cleaned him up. She said she had asked him if he was all right and he had said he was fine. "So," I said to the nurse, "Are you all right?' means "Do you need a bedding change because you have had a movement?" She said yes. I told her, "My husband, your patient doesn't understand the euphemism of your question. In addition, he no longer has sufficient sensation to feel a movement nor can he feel the wetness on his lower body. His only clues are gas pressure and odor."

Communication was a real problem at the hospital. Not only did a patient need to learn the language of medicine, a language rife with euphemism, there was also a literal language barrier within the staff. The majority of the nurses and aids on 6th floor oncology who cared for my husband were not native English speakers. This barrier often made it hard to understand questions and provide clear answers. To further compound the communication problem, this hospital is the only care facility where Fred was treated that required the patient to dial a nurse's cell number instead of using the nurse call button. The cell number was written on the wall using a dry erase board. The board was across the room from the patient. It is very hard for a bedridden patient to peer across the room then with a shaking hand to dial a cell number; let alone, use a clunky desk phone on a hard to reach side table. If a patient pushed the call button instead the patient was reprimanded by the nurses' station.

So my tasks grew ever larger in the kingdom of the sick. I would change Fred's bedding. I would walk to the nurses' station with our requests, as Fred stressed out about calling the nurse's cell phone number. I would get Fred's water and his ice.

I remembered the summer of 1976 and our family road trip. I rode the tallest Ferris wheel, and during that trip I would cherish the opportunity to get ice from the motel ice machine. I cannot pass a hotel ice machine without smiling. Have you ever noticed as an adult you must crouch down slightly to get ice from these machines? I have often thought they were designed with a child's height in mind. When I was four, many privileges and responsibilities were literally out-of-reach. I could not reach the sink to wash dishes or get a drink. I could not reach the dishes in the cabinets to set the table. But when we stayed in hotels, I began to relish my new duty of getting ice. I would take the ice bucket and would run down the hall to the ice machine. I would listen to its calming motor hum, as I would place the bucket on the lever. The rattling clunks would echo inside the machine, as the motor would gear up. The hole above the lever would begin to spew the mounds of ice into the bucket. Hotel after hotel, I would do this ritual and I discovered there were many types of ice. In some motels it would come out as cubes, sometimes it would be frozen rounded discs and sometimes wedge shaped smiles. By far, my favorite ice was the donut type. This ice would cascade out in circles. My sister, my brother and I would eat this ice like it was popcorn. I loved the way it would roll within my mouth. I would press my tongue until eventually the ice would turn thin and sharp, and then I would crunch my teeth upon the shards. I loved chewing ice, but even more I loved the ability to get that ice myself.

The child I was became the wife that stood in front of other ice machines. Pastel pitchers had replaced the old plastic bucket. I had lived much in the 33 years between hotel ice machines and hospital ice machines. I had married, given birth, managed stores and was well acquainted with both responsibility and privilege. So as I begged for access to information about Fred's diagnosis and treatment plan, I was handed a plastic pitcher and given a duty I could be trusted with. I could get him ice water. Each day, many times a day, I would get Fred ice. I would leave the room and carry that little pitcher down the hall and fill it up again and again. I grew concerned as time passed that the facilities did not replace nor clean the pitcher. In the first hospital we had the same pitcher for two weeks before it crashed upon the floor and shattered. It was then replaced. Fred went for another two weeks with his second pitcher.

So as Fred grew more ill, I often thought of ice and ice machines. The first thing I would do each day was to get him ice. The last task before leaving his room was to check and see if his pitcher was still filled. It made me sad. Sometimes I too, would drink the water and chew the ice. I would think of the ice I sucked upon while I labored before the birth of our two sons. I would think of the happy anxious father who would eagerly go down the hall to get me ice chips. He was so nervous he practically bounded down the hall. I smiled through the pain of childbirth, upon seeing his behavior, but at least that duty made him feel useful.

Little Miss A-Type Personality

WHEN FRED WAS IN THE hospital I spent weeks asking for information about his condition and getting very few answers. During the second week of hospitalization we desperately needed Fred's disability paperwork filled out for American University. Fred's oncologist rarely came to the room, so the social worker said she could fill most of it out for the doctor. The doctor became very angry that we had gone around him to get the paperwork completed. He was also angry that I was asking questions.

He went to my husband at 7:30am rounds and said; "I understand that your wife has been asking questions about your case." Fred said yes, with trepidation. Fred had worked in food service a great deal in his youth and knew exactly what happened to the hamburger of the customer who complained. Fred did not want me to cause trouble, because I went home at night and would not always be there to protect him. So Fred said yes, quietly agreeing his wife had been asking questions. The Doctor said, "Well, if Little Miss A-type Personality has questions, she should come to my office hours to ask them." When I arrived to Fred's room after I dropped the children off at school, he was very angry with me and worried that his care would be compromised because I had asked too many questions. I felt torn, between wanting to please my husband and knowing that something was going very wrong in his care.

The next day I went to the Doctor's office hours. I wore a church dress. The oncologist never closed the door in the fifteen minutes I had to speak with him. He never stopped taking phone calls, nor did he stop talking to the nurse who had her keys in hand as she complained about the parking problems in the employee lot. He discussed with a different nurse the transport and rooming arrangements of another patient by name. All the while I sat before him and waited. I was seated in a chair beside the trashcan. When he began to rattle off the points of metastasis at lightning speed, I said, "Please slow down because I don't understand all of these words. I am writing them down, so I can research them on the online."

He responded, "I don't like people who research on the online."

I said, "I am sorry but I don't have a background in medicine, so I have to research to understand what you are saying."

He said, "That is right, I am the one with the medical degree."

I looked up at him behind his computer screen. I looked at his medical degrees and awards on the wall behind him. On his right side were the degrees and his family portrait was on the wall to his left. I looked at his family portrait on the wall and I thought of our little family. He was shattering our family like glass in frame as it is thrown to the floor. We weren't an important part of his day. A moment that would change my life forever was only one more appointment in his over-scheduled workweek.

A doctor who wished to keep me small named me "Little Miss A-Type Personality." At the worst point of our life, this man named me a troublemaker. Did he want to drive a wedge in marriage that was 15 years long and would end only weeks later? Fred was sick and the oncologist in charge of Fred's case was as horrible as my father. I did not escape one tyrant so many years before to watch another let my husband die. I was forced once again into the role of a victim. We should not "complain" as it would only make it worse. We should wait in silence for a treatment that never comes. Only when the realization came that death was truly eminent, *when the gun began to spin*, would I be released from silence to secure our escape.

Not Just A Bad Doctor

Sometimes when I tell people Fred's story they want to resolve the tale with the statement: "You just had a bad doctor." I tell them no, we had a bad system of care and it must be fixed. When I left the office visit with Fred's doctor, I went back to Fred's room and he was missing. The nurses said he had just been wheeled down for an MRI. I found the MRI suite and the technician said I could wait with him until it was time for the test. Fred was very worried. He did not like tight closed spaces and this would be a long MRI experience. I drew my hand across his furrowed brow to soothe his troubled mind. He was hot to the touch. I asked the tech for a thermometer. The MRI tech said they did not have such tools in the MRI suite. I left Fred's side and went to the oncology ward and asked if someone could take his temperature, and failing that, could I borrow a thermometer and take his temperature myself. The nurses said they were too busy and there were no thermometers to spare.

I went back to Fred. He was hot and distraught. I managed to get him some ice water to drink. At this point the MRI technician grew concerned that Fred would not provide a good image if he did not calm down. I offered to go in with him to soothe him with my voice and presence. The technician said there was a policy to against allowing visitors in during the test. She called a nurse down from oncology to administer a second dose of Ativan. The nurse did not bring a thermometer though she did remark he was warm. She shot him with another dose of the anti-anxiety medication (my aunt Minnie, a retired ICU nurse later told me she would only give such a high level dose of Ativan to a patient who was actively violent prior to applying restraints.)

The tech wheeled Fred in and I told her I would be waiting right outside when she needed me. I waited for 15 minutes and the technician came out. She said she would not be able to do the test if Fred did not calm down. I followed her into the room. She told me to take off my ring and watch. I didn't know why she asked that; I just complied. I went over to hold Fred's feet. I began to shout soothing words over the railroad train roar of the MRI. Within moments my visitor ID tag tore off my blouse and shot across the room toward the MRI chamber. There it was lost. I had no idea how powerful the magnet was and could not grab the tag before it soared out of reach. I worried about it for a moment and then went back to the more pressing task of calming Fred. I yelled my love and endearments to Fred for over an hour. By the end I could barely speak and it was hard to hear, as I was not offered earplugs for the noise. But Fred got through the MRI and I had helped to calm him.

After the test, the tech paged a nurse again. Fred was very hot and his temperature was over 101 degrees. The nurse quickly tried to get approval for Tylenol while Fred was wheeled upstairs. Between the fever and the double dose of Ativan, Fred was altered in his behavior for the next 48 hours. He would not remember any events or the visits from friends that happened for the next two days. After diagnosis Fred only lived for 84 days. 48 hours lost may not seem like a big deal, but it is if you only have weeks left to live.

On April 9, 2009 Fred went back for two more MRI procedures. The entire process took about two hours. This time I stayed with Fred the entire time and the MRI technician offered earplugs. Fred was very tired and anxious after this additional test. Upon return to the sixth floor we told the transport we were supposed to go to the new room #6204 in

Oncology. The transport said he hadn't got new order so he would leave us in our old room on the general medicine side. Fred was in a great deal of pain at this point and needed to be hooked up to his PCA pump. I went down to the nurses' station. The general medicine nurse said it was not her responsibility as he was supposed to be moved to oncology. The oncology nurse said it wasn't her responsibility as we were not in our new room. When I went back to the room to tell this to Fred, he became very upset. I went back to the nurses' station and told them he would need his pain medications now. They said it was shift change and they would not be able to. At this point a nurse who was finishing her shift stepped in. She made both nurses come to the room. The two nurses and I moved the bed down the corridor without help from transport. When Fred got in the new room the pain pump was set up and was reengaged. I thanked the nurse who took charge of the situation.

On April 10, Fred's oncologist said he would like to begin radiation treatment for the bone metastasis. He asked Fred, "Would you like to do radiation treatment here or would you rather wait for a potential transfer to another hospital and do it there?" Fred asked what would radiation treatment accomplish. The doctor told him it would treat the bone pain. Fred hurt a great deal and said he would like to do "here" since he was already "here." We did not find out until later that day that we would have to go offsite to radiation.

An ambulance transport team entered our room in the afternoon. They were wearing full gear and had a collapsible ambulance gurney. With a clipboard in hand they said they would be transporting us to radiation. We did not understand. Fred said to them, "We were told we were having radiation here. I thought that meant downstairs." The crew replied, "No. Radiation is offsite. We have to transport you." I had never been part of a transport before, so I did not know what to do to help. One of the members of the team was new to the job and not fully certified. In the coming weeks I would learn the protocol of how to lift a patient from a hospital bed to a gurney. I would learn how to set the breaks, align the gurney, and carefully grab the pull sheet to lift the patient onto the gurney mattress. But on this day I did not know these things. The new technician had rarely dealt with patients who had bone metastasis. Instead of carefully lifting Fred she shoved Fred's hip. He yelled out in pain. She had shoved a point of metastases. When we secured transfer from that hospital two weeks later, x-rays would show Fred had broken his hip while bedridden.

Make-A-Wish

IN THE SPRING OF 2009, access to the internet was a reality for most homes in the United States. You could log on and Google a medical condition, post to friends on Facebook, and if you were really edgy you could even tweet. When my husband was diagnosed with probable kidney cancer within one day, I became a caregiver and a medical advocate. I would use the internet for both research and patient/family support. I, who swore to never own a cell phone, purchased one and used it daily to co-ordinate Fred's care. It wasn't a smart phone, but it helped a great deal. With no computer access in the hospital, I surfed the internet at night; researching his cancer using Google, reading the Wikipedia entry on kidney cancer with all of its links, and finding personal cancer stories. Facebook became our Caring Bridge, as we wanted an open community. I would take a few minutes each night to post to 100 plus people following Fred's care on Facebook. Within days of diagnosis, two of my friends had set up a *Lots of Helping Hands* account. This online network, which rapidly grew to 150 volunteers, would fundraise and provide meals, babysitting and groceries. This pool of helpers was immensely diverse. Before the creation of sites such as *Lots of Helping Hands,* orchestration of such a complex volunteer effort would not have been possible.

My husband was the model patient: he never complained or caused trouble. We were at the first hospital for four weeks with the only treat-ment being palliative radiation. My husband walked into that hospital, but soon he could no longer stand and could barely sit. We had no access to chemo or surgery nor did we have access to his electronic medical record. The hospital computer in my husband's room was broken. Nurses would have to leave the room to enter progress notes in Fred's record using the hallway computers. The nurses told us we were not allowed to use the hallway computers because they contained private patient data. The computer stations in the hallway faced the wall, limiting eye contact opportunities with the nurses. The nurses' station computer hub where the doctors would write orders was hidden behind frosted glass. When one of our guests visited, he used a hospital computer in the hallway unaware that he could access private patient data. He was able to surf the internet and check email.

During this confusing and frantic time we were using technology in a different way. When Fred was first admitted he could still stand and walk occasionally. There was a computer room for patients at the end of the hall. If he could walk down that hall, Fred could spend a few agonizing minutes surfing the web. He would post to friends and be himself in 12pt font. Soon he could not walk down the hall. Fred missed the access to the internet and the freedoms it entailed. Pain can be treated in many ways, with fentanyl, lidocain, and PCA pumps. But one of the best sources of pain relief for Fred was the internet: access to sites such as Facebook, IMDB, and *Ain't it Cool News*.

In February of 2009, Fred was talking a great deal about Stephen King's upcoming book, *Under the Dome*. He was so excited and researched it online. It would be a November release of a long awaited story. He briefed me on the tale. The concept of the book: a dome was encasing a small town in Maine and tensions were trapped within. This was a very special book. Fred said this book had been lost when the typed manuscript was left in a taxi cab years before. Stephen King had to rewrite the book from scratch. In March, Fred found out his pain was not the result of a slipped disk or muscle pull. His back hurt because of cancer in his spine. He lay in the hospital heartsick and imprisoned in a body and a bed. He turned to me and said, "What if I don't make it till November? I might not get to read *Under the Dome*."

Two days after he learned he had metastatic kidney cancer, Fred celebrated his 39th birthday in a hospital bed. On his feeding tray sat the hospital birthday cake, sparkling with ice and tasting of freezer burn. A friend gave him the comic book version of *The Stand*. Our younger son gave him a Dora the Explorer Balloon. I decided to try to get him the best gift ever. I could not stop his illness or get answers from his doctors. I could not walk for him or take his pain away, but I could try to get a galley copy of *Under the Dome*.

I emailed Deborah Johnson our wonderful book buyer at Child's Play, the toy-store where I worked. I asked her to please contact Simon and Schuster and see if it were possible to get a copy. She emailed her book representative Charlie. He contacted Tyler Le Bleu the marketing manager at Simon and Schuster. Tyler cleared the release with Stephen King. The book came on the perfect day. This was the day the oncologist said we could get surgery. With surgery Fred could live two more years! Two more years he would have to watch his sons grow older. In the midst of this rejoicing, I leaned over his bed like a princess in a fable and kissing him gave him the book. He was so happy he could not believe it. "I guess I'm really dying," he said. "I get my make-a-wish."

Thank God for that book. Fred took it on every radiation transport in the next two weeks. He read some everyday. The man, who could read a Stephen King book in less than 24 hours before he was sick, spent the next three weeks reading *Under the Dome*. While he was pinned in an MRI machine double-dosed with Adivan, I would scream the words of Stephen King at him above the train roar of the machine. Fred tried to read many books while hospitalized, but he only finished one: *Under the Dome*. I guess that makes a lot of sense, for it seemed like we living in a bubble. We were trapped in a hospital. I remember the one passage I read aloud to Fred. The character Brenda prays to God after losing her husband. "God, this is Brenda. I don't want him back...well I do, but I know You can't do that. Only give me the strength to bear this, okay? And I wonder if maybe...I don't know if this is blasphemy or not, probably it is, but I wonder if You could let him talk to me one more time. Maybe let him touch me one more time." That is when I burst in to tears and said to Fred, "I told you I would read to you, but how can I read that?" "It is okay, Reggie," he said. "I will read it myself." And he did.

I thank Stephen King for *Under the Dome.* I thank Tyler and Charlie and Deborah. This was a great good thing. Through this gift I would show Fred that I would do anything for him. This gift showed him there are many people who truly care. This book shined a light on our path of the beam, and we finished our love like we started it, talking Stephen King.

Prayers

DURING THIS DARK TIME OF Fred's first hospitalization, I prayed a lot. I thought a great deal about my past and the prayers that God had answered throughout my life. I would walk down daily to the hospital gift shop and look at the objects for sale that bordered between schmaltz and endearment. As I meditated upon crystals, rocks incised with words, and overly expensive Beanie Babies, I thought of all the years I worked at the Sapulpa Flea Market. It was hard, dirty work, and it made me despise at a very young age any passing fad or craze. Every couple years after a fad died the over-abundance of those products would crowd our stall and be almost impossible to sell.

To this day, I cannot stand termite shoes, Rubik's cubes, or feather earrings; but I truly utterly disliked the many mugs, wall hangings, and decorative pillows emblazoned with the words to "Footprints in the Sand." I found distasteful the hokey 1970's imagery of the beach sand and the disappearing footprints next to text written in mass-produced faux calligraphy. I am sure you are familiar with the tale. In it a man walks with God along a beach as the memories of his life pass him by. He notices in his darkest times there is only one set of footprints. He questions God, "Why did you leave me at my saddest moments?" God responds that when there was only one set of footprints that was when God carried him.

As a child, I really did not like "Footprints in the Sand." In many of the pictures accompanying the story, it seemed like Jesus was carrying the dead. The arms of the narrator were limp and dangling. I did not want to look at this and I did not want to be carried. Perhaps, as I was young, that memory of being carried, that loss of control or will was too fresh, so I could not accept this image. When I was a child, I spoke as a child; I understood as a child, I thought as a child. I remember the spring of 2009 when all things within this life seemed so very dark. I remember praying for the peace of God, that it fill me and uplift me and it did. I remember the exact moment. I was walking through the hospital cafeteria praying silently when I was filled with the love and light of God. My face was lit with an inner peace and even the hospital workers remarked upon my visage. The footprints artist had gotten it all wrong: when God carries you, you float.

As I write this book time has passed. I no longer burn with an inner fire. I smolder. The journey is long and I know the spirit is still within. I listen carefully and watch for "God moments." My sister Esther and I call moments of divine direction that happen with our lives "God moments." I listen, I am open to direction, and I know the freedom of putting one's life in God's hands. When Fred was sick, a lot of people said I should pray for a miracle. What they didn't understand is we already had a miracle.

Why did I watch *Doctor Who: Forest of the Dead?* I saw a relationship end in death, with a spouse powerless to stop it. That moment so moved me it changed our life. Fred and I watched the entire series in reckless joy. He said it felt like we were dating again, young again. I learned how helpful Facebook could be in organizing birthday parties or ... cancer care. I learned how to research The Doctor on the internet and would use that same knowledge to research real doctors on the internet. Do you remember Will Kemp, that Doctor Who fan from work? It turns out he could teach me how to create a blog called Regina Holliday's Medical

Advocacy Blog. Do remember Michael Wenthe? He was the friend whom we met at the faculty party and bonded over Doctor Who. He was the man who helped Fred home on the last day Fred attempted to teach class. Michael came to visit Fred every week without fail. He came to every hospital and to hospice and to home. He was with Fred the day before he died. He was the last friend Fred ever spoke to.

We were living our miracle.

Data Prison

TOWARD THE END OF APRIL I would learn there is a magical place in a hospital called the Medical Records Department. I would learn about this amazing place from a grief therapist. I was not sleeping very well. I spent most of my nights researching Fred's disease and most of my days at his side. I was so very tired. Friends offered to help with chores at the house and thereby relieve my workload. One day I left some plastic bins out for a friend so she could take the artistic things off my kitchen counter. In my mind's eye, I saw her placing my clay pots with their carefully sorted brushes and pencils neatly inside the plastic bins. This would enable other people to have more space to cook for the children. I came home to find all my supplies unceremoniously dumped together. Have you ever read that part in the Bible about the great wailing and gnashing of teeth? That adequately describes my behavior upon seeing my supplies buried this way. My mother-in-law Joan thought I had lost all sense of reason. Why was I screaming and weeping over art supplies, while my husband lay sick in the hospital? Why indeed, was I crying? I could not bear to lose them both. Not my husband and my art, that was too high a price to pay.

One of my friends thought I should see a grief therapist. I agreed to meet the therapist in her office, even though I wanted to speak to a medical librarian more than a therapist. I went to the therapist's office in the early morning prior to my day with Fred. I walked into a lovely peaceful room. There was a children's area with a little table and two little chairs. There was a wicker basket on the table filled with Sennelier oil pastels. I sat in a comfortable armchair across from the therapist. I recognized her as someone who had shopped at the toy store. I was somewhat antagonistic that morning and very tired. I stared at the basket of pastels as I told her that I didn't really need therapy. I needed access to Fred's medical record so we would know what was going on and decide on treatment options. She quietly asked me if I had tried going down to the medical records department. I broke my reverie with the pastel basket and glanced at her asking, "What is the medical records department?" She smiled a soft smile and explained it was the department in hospitals that kept all of the patients' medical records. If you requested patient records the medical records department would have to release them. I smiled and said thank you.

Then I rose from my chair and walked over to the basket of pastels. I gently pulled out a large red pastel. It was exquisite. The pastel was the finest you could buy. I asked her if she worked with children here, gesturing to the small table. She said yes, slowly rising from her chair with a smile. I asked her where she had purchased these pastels. She responded they came from an art store. She assured me they were artist grade and quite expensive. Nothing but the best materials would be provided for her young clients. I nodded in affirmation. I told her that I agreed the best materials lead to the best art, but *these were truly artist grade.* I held the pastel carefully touching only the paper wrapper and looked at her. I then said, "This pastel is a true cadmium red. It is a toxic pigment known to be a cancer-causing agent. The toxins can be absorbed through the skin, inhaled or ingested and lead to kidney cancer." She looked aghast. I continued looking down at the basket and placed the cadmium gingerly among its fellow colors, "I also see a viridian and a cobalt. They are toxic too. It looks like these have not been used yet, as all of their tips are still intact. I would highly recommend you remove them." The therapist quickly removed the basket from the table as I put on my jacket and headed toward the exit. I thanked her very much for her time and was very glad that I had taken precious moments to visit her. It looked like we both needed the other's advice.

On Friday, April 17, I went down to medical records to ask for a copy of Fred's entire medical record. There was a line of people trying to get information. There was an older couple filling out paper work to request a file. A couple with a young baby was next in line. Using a mixture of English and Spanish they managed to request the correct forms. I reached the counter and asked the clerk for a copy of my husband's entire medical record. As she pulled out the forms I would need, she said there would be a 73 cents charge per page for the medical record and a 21-day wait. I gasped. I said, "My husband is in this hospital right now on the sixth floor! All the information you need is in that computer. All you have to do is push print." She said that is just the way the system works. She handed me another form as she told me we would have to agree to all charges upfront. Even if there were duplicate pages or pages that appeared blank, we would pay 73 cents per page. I looked at her with disbelief and said, "My husband has been here for three weeks. That may be hundreds of pages." She responded that is just the way it is.

April 18, 2009 was a Saturday. Saturdays are quiet in hospitals. Few nurses walk the halls and most of the administration staff is gone, their offices dark and locked.

On Saturdays, I would stand by Fred's bed and wrap small presents for the children on the bedside tray table. We would hide these presents throughout the room for them to find on their Sunday visit. It was like an Easter hunt we had every week. On Sundays Isaac would sit next to Daddy's bed playing with toys. Sometimes Isaac would crawl up into Fred's bed. He would nestle there carefully within an embrace of arms and IV lines. As Fred's world grew smaller, and he could not stand nor walk; he just had room for Isaac. Isaac could lie beside him and cuddle. Isaac could still play silly finger games with Daddy. As Fred grew drawn and gaunt, Isaac would play Brio trains next to the catheter bag. Poor ten-year-old little Freddie would be so scared and sad he could barely look at Daddy. The hunt for presents was more for Freddie than for Isaac. Everything about the hospital disturbed Freddie. He could not tolerate the smells, the florescent lights, and the constant beeps of the alarms. He also had trouble regulating his voice and would often be admonished by the nursing staff for being too loud. One day as we left the facility, Freddie said, "Mommy, that hospital is like one of those blonde girls. The ones who seem so nice and pretty, until they open their mouth." These small presents helped make a bad experience bearable.

That Saturday morning the oncologist came to our door at 9:30am. He did not enter the room. He just stood in the threshold several feet away. He rarely visited so we had a list of questions ready in case he came by. The questions were taped to the bed so Fred would not forget them. We had five questions for him that morning: 1.When will Fred get a walker so he can walk again? 2. When will Fred be transferred? 3. When is surgery? 4. When will we get a pain consult? 5. When will we get chemotherapy? The doctor said we didn't need to worry about the questions. He said, "We've decided to send you home on PCA pump." I found out later that "we" meant the hospital, the oncologist, and the insurance company, aware of this decision days before Fred and I were. I had done my research. I knew exactly what was going on. This was home hospice. Fred was being sent home to die without being given a second opinion or access to his medical record. We were three weeks post diagnosis, stunned with tears pouring down our cheeks. We responded, "What about surgery? You said there would be surgery!" He just looked away from us and said, "There will be no surgery." I said "How can you just send us home? We live in a tiny one-bedroom apartment with two kids, one of them is three and the ten year old has autism. It is not even handicap accessible. How are you going to send us home?"

The oncologist said that would be a question for the discharge nurse on Monday. Then he turned his back and left us alone in a hospital on a Saturday.

In the business world they fire people on Fridays. There is a reason for that. They don't want people to make a scene. They don't want people to have access to open offices and be able to complain to the administration. After weeks of being told treatment was forthcoming, Fred's oncologist had the audacity to tell us we were going to home hospice without ever having the decency to say those words. My husband had gone along with every suggestion of this doctor up to this point. Now Fred turned to me and said defiantly, "Go after them Regina. Try to get me care." We had to suffer and wait that entire weekend, but on Monday I took action. I fired Fred's primary care physician that had never called nor visited. I asked my own primary if he would take on Fred as a patient. I thanked God that my doctor's specialty was geriatrics. He did not even pause before agreeing to take Fred on. He said, "After all, three of my current patients have kidney cancer." My doctor had privileges at another hospital and was instrumental in securing a transfer. I found a new oncology group that said they would see Fred. I spent three days organizing the transfer. Fred's nurse navigator from his insurance company was so frustrated by how hard it was to complete this transfer that she was crying to me on the phone. She said she would like to drive her Ford Explorer up to the front doors of the current facility and load him up herself. I told her to be calm; we had to do this the official way.

Later that day, the oncologist stormed angrily into Fred's room saying, "So you are transferring? Well no one will give you surgery." He left and I told the head nurse I wanted him barred from the room. Then I filed a complaint with customer service for his behavior and for the many ways Fred had suffered since being admitted. Next the internist warned Fred that this was not how things were done. The internist talked with Fred frequently and Fred really liked him. They were the same age, and both had three-year old children. I suppose I will call him Dr. Mango. Weeks before, I had begged him for in-depth information and he said that I was not behaving typically. I should be in a corner crying, like his wife would do if the situations were reversed. I stopped writing down notes. I said, "Dr. Mango, you really don't know anything about me. You don't know what has happened in my life and have no idea what I will do to protect the ones I love." Three weeks later as we prepared to leave the hospital, Dr. Mango came to see us. He told me the transfer didn't make any sense. We weren't going to a higher quality hospital. We were making a "lateral transfer." I said it did make sense, if you were trying to get a second opinion. Dr. Mango then shook his head sadly and went to sit with Fred. His shift was over and they talked about their children and the books they had read. Dr. Mango promised to visit Fred and said someday we would have a picnic with all of our children in the park. Then he left. Weeks later, when I sat by Fred's side, he turned to me and said, "Dr. Mango lied. He never came to visit. There will be no picnic." I could not help but think Dr. Mango has not had the kind of life experiences I have had. He has not suffered through the moments that teach you to be true, brave, and courageous. No matter how small or disempowered you are.

We were transferred on Wednesday, April 22, to the new facility. We were sent with incomplete and out of date medical record and transfer summary. That meant Fred was denied care for six hours while the nurses tried to cobble together a medical record using a phone and a fax machine. Without access to a current medical administration record, the nurses asked me questions about what kind of patches were on Fred and when were they placed? Both Fred's Lidocaine and Fentanyl patches weren't labeled or dated. Five days before I had begged for a copy of the medical record. If only it had been given to me, Fred would not have to suffer so. As the evening wore on the head nurse came to talk to me. She told me in her 20 years of nursing she had not seen such a screwed up transfer. She told me she was sorry because they could not even feed

Fred, as they had no dietary orders. She quietly told me there was a pizzeria downstairs. She said they *"would not see me"* if I went downstairs and got Fred a slice of pizza. A little before midnight an on call doctor gave Fred a basic examination so pain medication could be reinstated. Fred finally was calm and I went home to the children at 12:30 in the morning.

The next morning Fred's new oncologist shook his hand and sat beside him. This was such a wonderful thing. We had gotten used to a doctor who did not sit down and rarely touched his patients. Next my primary care physician came by and introduced himself also shaking hands with Fred. He said he would be watching out for Fred as a new patient to his practice, even though Fred would most likely not be able to come to the doctor's office. Fred's new doctors ordered an x-ray of his hip because Fred said it pained him so. Then the doctors took me aside and told me they wanted me to go back to the first facility in order to get a copy of Fred's entire medical record. I laughed at them saying, "I have been trying to get that medical record for four weeks. They will not give it to me." The doctors said, "They will give it to you this time. We're sending you as a courier. You are getting it for us." My mother-in-law Joan drove me over to the old hospital. The facility printed out the record in an hour and a half for the new doctors. I gave to them, along with all of Fred's films and CD's. The doctors looked at it for about an hour and then gave it back to me saying, "You should have this. You husband will be treated in many places, but if you have this you will be his continuity of care." I responded, "But you said this was important and you needed to read it." They replied, "It is and we did, but there isn't a place to put this in our computers. It is safest with you."

I read that record in 3 ½ hours. I spent the next few hours organizing the pages. I found so many mistakes and actionable data that had not been acted on. If I could have read the record on a daily basis his care would have been so much better.

The Horizon Line

My husband Fred had a favorite story about John Ford. Steven Spielberg told the tale. The story was an account of the day that Steven Spielberg met John Ford. The story went something like this. Steven was really young and had been making a few super 8 movies and he had the opportunity to meet John Ford in his studio. After waiting for about an hour, Mr. Ford came in and Steven Spielberg began to speak with him for a few moments. Mr. Ford said, "So, you want to be a picture maker." John Ford then gestured at a series of pictures on the wall. He asked Steven to describe what he saw. Steven started to describe the Native Americans and objects within the picture. That was not what John Ford was looking for. "No, no, " he said. "Where is the horizon?" Steven said that it was at the top of the frame. Mr. Ford asked Steven to describe the next picture. Again Steven began describing the Calvary and elements, and again Mr. Ford was frustrated. "No, no. Where is the horizon?" Steven looked and said, "It is at the very bottom of the painting."

John Ford said "When you are able to distinguish the art of the horizon at the bottom of a frame or at the top, but not going right through the center of the frame, when you are able to appreciate why it is at the top and why it is at the bottom, you might be a pretty good picture maker. Now, get out of here." That is a great story and Fred would tell it to his college film students, and I would tell it to my pre-k art students for years to come. I loved that story because it makes it very clear that the angle from which you view things has an effect on how you see things. As a family caregiver for my husband, my view was a limited one. I knew about ice chips, bedding changes, and bed sore prevention. I was educating myself each night but my learning curve was steep. As I spread Fred's medical record before me, I saw the world of medicine from a very different angle. Fred had told me he only had a three-centimeter tumor in his kidney. He misheard the doctor. He had a three-centimeter tumor in his sacrum. If my husband and I could have seen the written results of the CAT Scan/Bone Scan/ MRI we could have had reached an understanding of the scope of his disease so much sooner. The oncologist gave a verbal diagnosis to a patient alone. Fred had tried to remember the words he was told. He told me the oncologist said a three-centimeter tumor in left kidney and a cyst in the right. The actual dimension was a nine-centimeter tumor in right kidney and 6.6-centimeter mass in left kidney. The mass in his abdomen was huge. It was creeping up and through his inferior vena cava like the taproot of some monstrous dandelion. What we had here was a failure to communicate.

The most glaring example of inaction was Fred's distended bladder. When Fred was admitted on March 25, his intake form specified a history of urethral stricture. Fred's MRI of his pelvis that day stated, "Bladder appears distended suggesting retention." On March 28 the bone scan results specified "Urinary bladder markedly distended making evaluation of the sacrum and low lumbar spine impossible." All the while my husband was fighting a fever due to infection, and the nurses are not sure where the infection was coming from. On April 4, the nurse's progress report mentions a concern about urine retention.

The CAT scan of April 10 stated, "Place catheter for extremely distended bladder." This scan was done at the offsite radiation facility, the day of our first ambulance transfer; the day Fred most likely suffered a metastatic break to his hip. The radiologist came over to me after Fred's scan. She firmly grasped my shoulder and said, "Mrs. Holliday, I have tried calling your husband's doctor. I have tried calling the hospital. No one is returning my calls. Your husband has a dangerously distended bladder and it is interfering with imaging results. You need to make sure a catheter is placed as soon as you return to the hospital." Fred and I returned via ambulance transport. As soon as Fred was in his bed, I went to the nurses' station. I told the head nurse about the radiologist's concerns. I said, "Fred must have a catheter placed immediately, but I need to let you know he has a pre-existing condition called an urinary tract stricture. He has had a catheter placed twice in life and both times a urologist was needed." The nurse said they would try anyway. First they tried with a 16 gauge and were unsuccessful. Then they tried with a 12 gauge and were unsuccessful. They gave up. Fred's oncologist ordered a urology consult for the next day. Finally the urologist placed a catheter, 17 days after the medical record deemed it necessary. The progress notes from the day before stated that *Fred had refused treatment.*

I was filled with righteous anger. That was a lie. Fred went along with everything that they asked of him. He was incredibly compliant. The hospital staff had not acted appropriately and in a timely fashion; they had not read his medical record. They were blaming the victim, when the fault lay with them. I had read Fred's medical record and I organized it. It was now contained in a binder that was 3-inches thick. I had highlighted errors and amended progress notes with revisions that better reflected reality. I brought this tome to the nurses' station at our new hospital and I asked a nurse, "Who reads the medical record?" Her response was, "We read the face sheet and maybe the most recent pages. No one reads the entire record."

The Second Hospital

EVERYONE WAS VERY NICE AT the second hospital. The staff listened and they were helpful. They answered questions and assigned a cancer care navigator to Fred. They even had a massage therapist that came once a week to offer a foot massage to every cancer patient. The technicians performed bedding changes with great care and talked to Fred as though he were a person not a placeholder.

In the oncology waiting room at the second hospital, the light was on. It was serene and smelled of flowers and fresh chocolate chip cookies. The television, with intact channel buttons, was mounted within easy reach. The remote control was set upon a table bedecked with flowers. The staff and visitors often gathered and chatted with the families. Every Wednesday afternoon there was a tea at two o'clock. Patients, visitors, and support staff congregated as fresh chocolate chip cookies were passed around. This room was filled with smiles and laughter; the burden of grief was lessened by the support of others.

An organized display shelf of educational pamphlets written by the National Cancer Institute was placed beside the door. Within this display, there was a book devoted entirely to kidney cancer. Beside the pamphlets, another rack was filled with inspirational tracts with names such as "You have the Right to Be Hopeful" and "A Time to Live." All these elements created a feeling of hope and choice within this hospital. I know my father would have looked at all of these fine things and smiled his crooked smile. He would have said, "You can kill a cat with kindness, too."

Within days Fred's new doctors wanted to do surgery, but this wasn't the de-bulking surgery that had been recommended at our prior hospital. The new hospital determined that Fred indeed did have a broken hip. They recommended surgery to "pin" the hip. I questioned this recommendation. I said, "Fred had stopped walking prior to breaking his hip. He's been in pain for a long time and bedridden for over a month. How will this surgery help?" The doctors told us the only way we would get debunking surgery that might extend Fred's life was if Fred could walk again. The only way he could walk again was if they fixed his hip. Surgery was scheduled and I went down with Fred to the surgery suite. There they had a ream of paperwork for Fred to sign agreeing to the procedure. After Fred affixed his signature, they asked him if he had any questions. Fred said, "Yes, how big is the 'pin' you are placing in my hip?" The surgeon chuckled and said, "Oh, it is not a pin, think of it as a piece of rebar being shoved inside your leg. After this when you get a x-ray it will look like there is an erector set inside of you." Fred was wheeled into surgery and Joan and I waited anxiously in the lobby.

Fred's hip surgery was successful and he was sent to recovery. Like any patient who has had a knee replacement or a hip pinned, the staff wanted to get Fred up as soon as possible. The physical therapist came to our room and tried to get Fred to stand. He screamed instead. His sacrum was a point of metastasis as well and there isn't a pin for that. The therapist gave me instructions for bed exercises and then made sure compression sleeves were placed on Fred's legs, as she was very concerned about potential blood clots.

In our second week of hospitalization at the new facility and the sixth week since our initial admission, we still had not received chemotherapy drugs. I asked our nurse navigator why the drugs still had not arrived. She found out the hospital pharmacy had repeatedly kicked out the order, as it was too expensive. She told me I would have to order it myself and she would fax in the prescription. She gave me the number for a specialty pharmacy that allowed us to order Fred's Sutent. The pills would be mailed to my apartment building; the front desk would have to sign for the package. I would have to bring the drugs to the hospital myself. The 28 pills cost $40,000.00.

Minutes Of Sunshine

Do you remember the little red wagon of your youth? I remember mine. I remember the rusty grit of the metal and the embossed grove design on the bottom of the carriage. I remember the wagon was an excellent tool in which to pile fall leaves or dozens of pecans from the tree in our backyard. If my sister Esther and I sat cross-legged we both fit within the wagon as our brother pulled us down the sidewalk. But I would squeal for joy when I could lay down alone in the bed of the wagon and my brother would pull me along. The clouds would race in the sky above me and my hair would ripple across my face as we careened down the sidewalk. It felt like flying. The ride would never last long though. My brother was only a child himself and could only pull at racing speed for minutes, but how I cherished those minutes of sunshine.

When my husband Fred was sick he was not pulled in a red wagon. He was lifted onto a gurney and strapped in place 46 times for transport. He was rolled out of hospital doors and into ambulances where EMS teams would transport him for radiation or other treatment. I did the math once and realized that Fred experienced an accumulated three hours of sunshine and fresh air during his eleven weeks of hospitalization due to transport.

After the hip surgery at the second hospital, Fred's doctors said they needed to begin radiation again. Fred had already finished a 10-day course of radiation at his prior hospital that focused on his lower back. This time they needed to focus on his leg, as the surgery to "pin" his hip would have pushed cancer cells deep into his leg. So once again Fred would begin daily bed to gurney transfers and leave the facility with full ambulance support.

Fred was sick during the spring in Washington, DC. If you have ever been to DC in the spring, you know the city is bedecked with flowers. I remember during transport after transport the blossoms would gently fall upon the gurney, as the EMT would push through the doors of the radiation facility. Then the EMT team would leave us in the hall. Gurneys would line the hallway like cattle in their stalls. I would stand by Fred and hold his hand as strangers and technicians would brush by us as they headed to the waiting room or the radiation suite. Fred would close his eyes and avoid the stares of strangers and the fluorescent glare of the blinking lights of above. He would wait and suffer until it was time for transport again, until it was time for falling blossoms and minutes of sunshine.

Our days became a series of physical therapy exercises, attempts to sit up, and transports for radiation. Each night I would continue to research and grow more and more concerned. It seemed like we were on some kind of evil roller coaster ride. Fred's various symptoms were being treated but not his body as a whole. The more I researched his condition and compared it to his medical record the more I worried about his prognosis. The more I researched disease in patient populations the more I worried about our entire medical system. Too many people were suffering in the dark. Too many people were grasping at minutes of sunshine while falling into the shadows.

On April 29, I sent an email blast to everyone I knew. I was appalled at the care patients receive: the lack of access to data and the lack of coordination of care. I had worked retail since the early 1990s. Who has heard of a decent-sized store that doesn't have a computerized point of sale system? What business provides service without an itemized receipt? I have yet to find a store that charges the customer for their copy of that receipt. I had been a special education advocate for my son since kindergarten. I had been part of many IEP meetings and had read reams of test results, as was my right under the Freedom of Information Act. But in my role as caregiver and patient advocate, medical records personnel told me if I wanted a copy of Fred's medical record I would have to pay 73 cents a page and wait 21 days. How can a patient or caregiver be part of the team if they have no access to that data? In my email blast I spoke of all those families and patients who suffer in silence. I said we must change this very broken system.

On Saturday, May 2, 2009, at 12:39 AM I wrote a second email to all my Friends and this time I had a plan:

> *Dear Friends, Business Associates, Special Ed/Educational Contacts, & Artists,*
>
> *Most of you are aware that my husband, after two months of fruitless Doctors' visits and two trips to two ER's, was diagnosed with Stage IV Kidney Cancer on Friday March 27th, 2009. We plunged into the nightmare that is modern medical care in the USA. I found out I needed to be with my husband constantly to make sure we received even basic care. We were going to be released to home or institutional hospice after a month of only palliative treatment. We fought for transfer to another hospital for a second opinion. We are now getting treatment. This has been a horrible experience.*
>
> *The more I talk to other people the more I hear the same story. "The doctor did not listen." "The nurse did not read the chart." "The hospital kicked us out because insurance was*

running out." It goes on and on. I ask all these wonderful people what did they do to right this injustice? The response is the same. "I was too tired." "It was too hard." "I was so sad." "They just got away with treating us this way."

This has to stop. This is not right.

Why do we have more transparency in Special Education law then in Medical Care? Why do we have more access to information on a Box of Cheerios then on a medical chart? Why do medical records personnel think the Freedom of Information act does not apply to them? We need to do something. The system is broken. It is up to us to fix it.

People tell me just concentrate on your husband, your family. Too many people have quietly done that. Too many wonderful fathers, mothers and children are gone. Too many graves have flowers on them. I will fight. I will not stop. I will not be silenced.

Today I had an Epiphany. You might have seen my mural work on the side of the American City Dinner. I painted all those Famous Stars from the 30's through the 50's about six years ago. I also painted the mural of the children reading at Child's Play. I painted the St. Jude's Hospital Thanks and Giving mural on the old Hechts Building about five years ago. I would like to do a new mural series.

I want to do a Medical Advocacy series. I am doing a design based on the Food packaging "Nutrition Facts" Label. Instead of Nutrition Facts, it will be "Medical Facts Mural." I want do a Simple Anatomy Drawing that highlight's the patients illness. To the side of this will be an easy to reference list of all pertinent info. This will be done in such a way as to mimic a Nutrition

Label. I think this will be very eye-catching. I want senators and congressmen, bus drivers and waitresses to drive by this and want this kind of clarity and transparency for themselves.

Where do you come in? I need walls. I would prefer them white primed and ready for mural work. And I want these murals be in the busiest areas of Washington, DC.

I may be only a mother, a wife, a sales girl, a teacher, an artist, and a caregiver; but I will effect change. I will give all my talent, my abilities, my energy, and my belief to helping us all. Someday you will not have to fear a trip to the hospital. You will know you will be cared for. No wife or husband will have to fight the silent fight for the one they love. I will stand up. They will take notice. I will never give up.

Please forward to this to anyone you think could help.

Thanks for your time,
Regina Holliday
(The really nice lady at Child's Play)

Most of the people who read this email, commiserated with my pain and helped in other ways, but a few people offered up walls. A friend who worked in a basement massage parlor said they had some space, but it was determined that they had little foot traffic there. The owners of Pumpernickel's Bagelry and Delicatessen on Connecticut Avenue said they had about 5'x6' of space in the deli. Fred and I had eaten off and on at Pumpernickels for 15 years. They were fast and efficient. The food was good and fresh. The dining space was very small, like in many establishments in the city. The staff did not suffer fools lightly; but they were incredibly kind when incredible kindness was needed. The owners, Rob and Brigid Gillette, said I could use the space right beside the menu. I asked them, "Are you sure? I am going the paint end-stage cancer right next to bagels and lox." They said that they were sure; they wanted to help, as they had seen their own family suffer in hospitals. It was a very kind and selfless act. That painting was on the wall for four years and helped create better health policies for us all. Pumpernickel's has grit. It has grit on floor from the shoes of the hundreds of dedicated local fans and grit of spirit.

Jamie Crausman, a friend of Fred's from his years pursuing his Master degree at American University, also reached out to me. He said he had no walls to donate but he did run a small editing company. He said he and his team would film the mural that I painted.

Sanity Shifts

ON MAY 3, 2009, I worked a short shift at the toy store. I worked three days while Fred was sick. I called them "sanity shifts." For a few hours, I left the hospital. For just a short while, I was not the wife of that poor young father recently diagnosed with cancer. I went back to working retail in order to reclaim some semblance of normal, but as I sold toys to parents and answered questions about art projects, my heart beat within my ears and I could find no peace. At closing time, a customer whom I had helped for many years came in. It was Christine Kraft. I felt compelled to talk to her. The air around us was electric. It was meant to be. We barely knew each other. I was the nice shop-keep. She was the nice customer. I stopped her and said, "I feel I must tell you that my husband has stage 4 kidney cancer." I had no idea at the time, but Christine is what one would call an internet maven. She connects people. She looked at me and her eyebrows raised and her mouth opened. She said, "I was just at a medical conference and I met this amazing man ePatient Dave! He had stage four kidney cancer and survived!" I excitedly responded, "He survived stage four kidney cancer? Almost no one survives stage four! I must meet this ePatient Dave! How do I find him?" Christine said I would have to get on twitter. I responded, "What's the twitter?" Christine just smiled, hugged me and said go home and Google it tonight.

With the help of my ten-year-old autistic son I learned how to log onto twitter. I sent my first tweet on May 3 at 11:10 pm: "I am trying to talk with Christine Kraft and epatient Dave." Now, if you know anything about twitter, you know I did that wrong. But Dave is so amazing he found me from that tweet. He tried to respond via twitter and realized quickly I was twitter incompetent. Dave then contacted me via email. That night I learned about the term e-patient. I learned about ACOR (Association of Online Cancer Resources). I had been doing research for eight weeks but had never found this special list serve called ACOR. I would converse via email with the list founder Gilles Frydman and would see post after post from people across the world fighting cancer. I joined the kidney cancer sub-group and saw so many people were attacking this disease with methods that had never been suggested by our oncologists. These people on the list serve were all so very hopeful.

Dave then called me on the phone to explain what had happened to him. ePatientDave used to be a regular guy with a regular name. He was born in 1950 and named Dave deBronkart Jr. He worked for many years in multiple industries before becoming a member of the IT movement in 1989. In January of 2007, he was diagnosed with metastasized renal cell carcinoma stage four. Most patients die within months of this diagnosis and there is a less than 5% survival rate for the two years following diagnosis. Dave, as an experienced Internet researcher, used every search engine at his disposal to research and help decide the treatment options for his disease. He and his collaborative physician decided on laparoscopic surgery and he participated in a clinical trial of high-dose interleukin-2. The dual treatment was successful and he is now cancer free. His whirlwind experience in trying to get the correct treatment within a short time window informed his choice to take a new life path. Dave was becoming a public speaker and blogger on patient empowerment, participatory medicine, and patients' rights.

As I talked with Dave I was making macaroni and cheese for dinner. My three-year-old son Isaac was constantly wrapping his arms around me as I cooked and trying to talk. The poor little boy was so starved for time with Mommy in this the seventh week of his father's hospitalization. As I danced around the kitchen balancing both motherhood and patient advocacy, the phone cord spiraled around both Isaac and me. As I told our story to Dave, I looked down at my phone cord bondage. It seemed like I was being embraced by hundreds of the little letter "e."

Next Dave wanted me to speak with his doctor. By late that evening Dave's oncologist from Harvard, an authority in kidney cancer, was calling me to talk about Fred's prognosis. Dave's doctor listened while I explained his current state of disease. He did not interrupt as I listed procedures and protocols. I had tried to speak with other doctors who were friends of our family about Fred and get their opinions. They always responded that they could not really comment unless they examined Fred. Dave's doctor listened intently and then he did a very brave thing. He responded to my questions. He quietly told me the ACOR kidney cancer group could be quite helpful to many people, but Fred's cancer was very advanced based on the information I had shared with the doctor. There was a pause on the line then he said, "Sometimes we catch these things too late. Sometimes there is nothing we can really do. Sometimes the best thing you can do is to decide how to spend the life you have left."

Blue

ON MAY 6, 2009, I got a call at 7:30 in the morning from Fred's old primary care physician's office, the one who had given pain medications
rather than a diagnosis. It was the physician's assistant. She was calling
to tell me that the oncologist from our first hospital had warned them
I might be making waves. I could not believe they were calling us now.
"Waves?" I responded. "If by waves you mean that you are wondering if
we will sue you, the answer is no. If waves mean I will do everything in
my power to change national health policy and improve the system of
care in the United States, then that is a yes. And by they way you should
always weigh your patients, as massive weight loss is a sign of cancer."
Click.

Within two days it was time to leave the second hospital. They
said they had done all they could. Fred would need to walk again
before more could be done. The doctors said Fred would need to go
to a rehab facility to regain his walking ability. On May 8, 2009, Fred
was transferred to a rehab facility deep in Maryland. We were placed
there so Fred could learn to walk again after being bed-ridden for six
weeks. Fred had metastasis of the lower spine and pelvis. He had also
suffered a metastatic break to his left hip that was pinned via surgery.
He was undergoing a second series of radiation and had just begun
chemotherapy. In order to transfer to rehab, Fred had been taken off
his PCA pump and his oral steroids, as those methods of pain control

were not possible in rehab. Fred had been placed on Percocet instead and was in excruciating pain.

Fred had made friends with a great many staff members at the second hospital and many of them said goodbye. On our last evening our favorite bed change technician came by. She was a very kind heavy-set woman with most beautiful hair weave consisting of flowing ringlets of tight curls. She said she had heard we were transferring to rehab. She asked where we were going. We told her the name of the rehab center and the smile dropped from her face. She told us they were woefully understaffed and often low on supplies. She went to her supply cart and began placing package after package of adult cleaning wipes and rubber gloves in a big bag. She tied it off and gave it to me saying, "You will need this."

Fred grew weaker and weaker at rehab. The staff removed his compression cuffs. They said he would not need them as he *"was going to start walking soon."* He tried so hard to walk in rehab, but it was almost impossible. On his best day he managed six steps and then never walked again. The rehab had been designed for post-surgery and accident victims not end-stage cancer. It was a place where pain was good. Fred tried so very hard to work with his physical therapist and she knew he did. She would visit most days when no one else would. By the second week she was the one who discovered Fred had a blood clot that stretched from his surgery incision point to his knee. All physical therapy and unnecessary movement of his leg was stopped and Fred was given blood thinners.

The oncologist only visited for 15 minutes in the two weeks Fred was in rehab. We had chosen this facility so far from our home because the oncologist said he would visit us here. The doctor in charge on the floor was studying for his boards and seemed genuinely frightened of Fred's stage of disease. There was one nurse for 20 patients and few techs for bed changes. After all, you were supposed to walk to the bathroom in rehab. The sinks were too shallow to fill a washing basin. I asked the staff how did they accomplish a full body wash. They responded that patients were supposed to go to the showers. If they could not, they would be washed with the few cups of water that could be poured within the basin.

This was a place where you were supposed to eat in the cafeteria, and if you stayed in your room you were punished. You were fed last. Fred feebly joked, "Based on the quality of food he had seen so far, not eating is a pleasure not a punishment." Joan and I would drive to all the local fast food places and get hamburgers and milk shakes, anything to tempt Fred to eat. Fred could barely sit up in his bed let alone stand. But he tried so hard.

We paid extra so Fred could have a private room in rehab. Like the Little Princess in her attic, I tried to make this scary place beautiful. I turned the spare bed into a type of sofa with a liberal application of throw pillows, well-tucked sheets and blankets. We rearranged the chairs for our infrequent guests, for Fred had been in the hospital for over seven weeks now and the flood of visitors had become a trickle.

On Fred's walls were mostly paintings I would kindly call "motel art." Many hospitals and hotels place insipid paintings on their walls. In attempt to please everyone, they please no one. Fred really disliked the one print that depicted a cow in a field by a barn. He said he did not want to sleep with that cow looking at him. I moved it to the far wall, blocked from view by the sink area. The other walls were bedecked with landscapes and seascapes. They were flat paintings, not at all the kind of pictures you could fall into. They did not have the depth of emotion that a true artist can depict, even if that artist is a child.

For seven years I taught pre-school students landscape and seascape painting. Many parents framed their children's inspired depictions of nature. Before beginning seascapes, I reminded them of the summer landscapes we did. I said, "In a summer landscape the sky is blue, and it is the top part of your picture. The bottom part of your picture is grass and it is green. The grass and sky meet and form the horizon line at some point in the painting." The kids chorused along with the words blue and green as I spoke. "Today we will do a seascape. The sky will be …" "Blue," chorused the children's sweet voices. I smiled upon them and continued, "and the sea will be …" They paused for a moment and shouted, "BLUE!" Then they burst into giggles, because even they knew you would not see the horizon line if everything were blue. We all laughed for a moment and then I began to explain there are many types of blue…

There are indeed many types of blue.

May is the month I was born. It is the month of Mother's Day. It is the month for rummage sales. It is the month I began to blog and that I placed the first painting in the Medical Advocacy Mural Series. It is the month Fred agreed to go to Hospice. This month means many things to me, and a few them make me feel blue.

I always looked forward to May. As a small child, my neighbor, Mrs. Johnson would cut a large bouquet of peonies as a gift for my birthday. I so looked forward to those flowers. I looked forward to the cards that would come from my aunts and uncles. I anticipated the joy of celebrating my birthday. I remember the day itself was never quite as wonderful as the anticipation of the day. I loved looking forward to things. I still do. I am constantly involved in projects that I spend weeks or months visualizing and anticipating. Oh, I love them when they are complete, but the true joy is in the anticipation of the process. This is the breathless excitement of a child at Christmas, the anticipation of joy.

So with great confidence, I can say there is no worse grief than anticipatory grief. This is the grief that drags you down and runs like a

24-hour movie in your mind. This is the grief that makes the last days with your loved one not bittersweet, but anguished. It almost feels like you have turned into a computer with two programs running and those two programs are diametrically opposed to each other.

Why did I beg Fred's doctors for his records? For the first time in my life, I desperately wanted to be wrong. From what little information I had gathered combined with my research, I knew Fred had only a few months to live. I vividly remember Fred's hospitalist telling me I was not behaving typically as I beseeched him for a prognosis. I should be crying and in denial, as he assured me his wife would be if our situations were reversed. I read about the stages of grief: denial, anger, bargaining, depression and acceptance. I went through these stages at a soul crunching speed during Fred's illness. I loved him so and cared for him daily and accepted in my heart of hearts he was dying. I felt schizophrenic in my love. My mother-in-law Joan was so angry with me. How could I accept this? I remember posting the "Get Well, Soon" cards on Fred's wall with such a sense of sorrow. I remember feeling like I was living a lie every time I accepted someone's well wishes. I was splitting into two and I wore a mask to hide my sorrow. Of all the types of blue, I do think anticipatory grief is the hardest to cope with. This is grief that is very lonely. You are the crest of the wave and everyone else is so far below and it so very frightening to know soon you will crash upon the shore.

In May of 2009, my birthday fell on Mother's Day. Fred and I joked over the years that he didn't have to buy me many presents as our anniversary was the day after Christmas and my birthday was so often on Mother's day. Sundays were the days we took the boys to visit Fred while he was hospitalized, so we would celebrate my birthday in Fred's room at the rehab center. Christine Kraft made me a chocolate cake with 37 pink and green striped candles. It was wonderful cake that tasted like the ones Aunt Hilda used to make. I cut Fred a slice and we all got in my mother-in-law's car for the drive to the rehab center.

When we got there, Fred's eyes were focused on the ceiling. There was a hornet in the room. We had already been dealing with ants coming in through cracks in the window caulking and now it was wasps. I went down to the nurses' station to complain and ask for assistance. The nurses said they would send a janitor. I tried to get the hornet myself, but I was so short I could not reach it. We waited 45 minutes and no one came. The cleaning staff had left for the day. I went back to the nurses' station and asked for help. The nursing supervisor came. She stood on a chair and tried a few sweeps with a newspaper. She only succeeded in making it mad. She then got off the chair and told me she couldn't get it and needed to go back to the nurses' station. She left and my family looked at me. My husband looked at me in resigned defeat. My two little boys looked at me with the fear little ones reserve for flying stinging things. My mother-in-law just stared.

I picked up a Newsweek Magazine with the Starship Enterprise on the cover and began to climb. I climbed on chairs and bedside tables swatting at that wasp. I chased it around the room. How dare it invade our fragile peace? How dare it worry my husband who was lying in a bed he could not arise from? How dare it scare my children who would only see their father for a few hours tonight? I climbed and swatted. Finally, climbing across the guest bed sofa, I hit it. It fluttered its last and fell to the floor. My eldest son Freddie let out a whoop. Three-year-old Isaac laughed a joyful giggle. I spun around with them in the center of the room as we did a happy dance. Fred looked on with a smile. We had killed the wasp. We could do this one thing to make a horrible time a little better. After our giggles subsided, we stayed a few hours and talked. Fred never ate his piece of cake; he did not feel much like eating.

Transitions

ON SATURDAY MAY 16, 2009, I was with Fred in his room. My sister Esther had come for a short visit. She was home with the children, and Joan had gone back to Grantsville for a very short break from life at the hospital. Every once in a while we all needed our "sanity shifts." I had brought my painting supplies with me and painted beside Fred on the rice paper sheets that would soon make the painting "The Medical Facts Mural." I looked much like the day Fred first met me 17 years before. I knelt on the floor painting, my hair pulled back with a paintbrush in hand. I was even using the same brushes. I looked up at Fred, smiling, ready to share this memory, but he was sleeping. He had been sleeping most of the day; I began to worry that he might need a blood transfusion. I pulled out his medical record and counted the days between transfusions. He had had a transfusion about every 14 days. Today was day 15 or 16.

I brought the medical record with me to the nurses' station and asked for a stat CBC. She looked at me and said the tech had already left the facility for the day and would not be back till tomorrow morning. I showed her Fred's record and again expressed my concerns. She said she would ask a tech to come over from the hospital. The hospital was less than 50 yards away on the other side of the parking lot. The tech arrived within two hours, blood was drawn and the lab results did show that Fred was in need of a transfusion. "Okay, when do we begin the transfusion?" I asked. "Oh, we don't do that here," said the nurse. "You will have to get him transferred to a hospital, and that won't happen till Monday because we are understaffed." Did I mention the hospital is less than 50 yards away?

At this point we had done over 40 ambulance transports. An amazing company called Team Critical Care did the last 20 transports. The company had been created as a ground service transport for critically ill patients as a complement to helicopter service. They were dedicated and well trained. I carried their phone number with me everywhere I went. I called them up and asked what paperwork was needed for a hospital transfer with ambulance support. They told me what was needed, and I went back to the on duty nurse. I asked nicely for the needed papers for the ambulance team. She printed them out and then I asked for my own copy. She said, "We don't do that." I told her I understood that she was not supposed to give me my own copy, but couldn't she do it secretly in our room? After all, I was very aware of the dangers of lost paperwork during transfer. She gave me my own packet, and as the nurse left our room she warned me that if we did not return within 24 hours we would lose our room at rehab.

The ambulance arrived and we were driven across the parking lot. We were admitted through the ER and waited six hours to get a bed. When we got up to the floor, I asked to see his inpatient medical administration record. I compared it with my own copy. The hospital had an error on the dosage amount on a drug Fred was taking. I pointed it out to the doctor. She was very nice and immediately corrected the record. The room was a shared one with another male patient, but the doctor let me stay with Fred through the night as he was transfused. The night nurse thanked me profusely, as I did all of Fred's bedding changes myself. The next morning was Sunday. I asked about transport back to rehab. The staff person at the nurses' station told me "Good luck with that, we have 70 patients to discharge and one discharge nurse on duty."

So I called Team Critical Care once again, and once again they talked me through the process of gathering all the necessary papers. Thank God for Team Critical Care.

We transferred back to rehab with one hour to spare. The staff was already packing up our belongings, as they knew weekend transfers were almost impossible. Usually, after transfusion Fred was happy and rosy cheeked, but not this time. He was tired and he still pallid. As I sat with him that morning I was exhausted. I wondered what would happen next. Within a few hours, the doctor who had overseen Fred's transfusion in the hospital came over to the rehab. She was very concerned. After her shift was over she felt she must talk to me about Fred's condition. Fred didn't really belong in rehab; he belonged in hospice she quietly told me. She said I would need to get the oncologist to write the hospice orders. The rehab discharge staff could handle the paperwork. I thanked her for her kindness in stopping by. Then she left to go home and get some rest.

I looked over at Fred with tears in my eyes. It was time for another transfer. Soon Fred awoke. He looked so very tired. I told him what the doctor said. Tears pooled in his eyes. He said, "I guess it is time to give up. It's time to die." When we filled out Fred's Advance Directive at the first hospital, we did it all alone. Tears ran down my face as I read question after question to my newly diagnosed husband. We had never even spoke of this in theory; we had never practiced. There was no one to help us answer the questions on that form. Now we had to answer the questions again. Again I sat alone with my husband, his eyes as trusting as a child, while I explained the DNR forms that must be signed before transport to hospice. I stood steadfast at his side supporting his decisions and I was thankful the family united around him with the goal of a good and peaceful death.

Soon the discharge supervisor came to our room. She was still await-ing the transfer orders from the oncologist. They wanted Fred's bed for another client and were getting impatient. I had called the oncology practice several times and left messages but the doctor had not called back. Later that afternoon, the local doctor who oversaw Fred's blood transfusion called. She asked if the oncologist had been reached. I told her he had not answered my calls. She exhaled a long-suffering sigh, and then asked for his number. She told me she was sure he would take a call from another doctor. She got approval in five minutes.

A few days later Fred's oncologist called me back. I was in the toy store parking lot having just picked up toys for the children. It was a windy day and my hair whipped around my face as I held the phone in one hand and my bags in the other. I spoke to the doctor and told him Fred was failing fast. He responded that hospice had always been an option. It was always a choice. At this point, I was very mad at the nice oncologist. He had shaken hands with Fred. He had been so kind; yet he had recommended a hip surgery that was pointless. He had recommended a rehab that he had never visited and a treatment protocol that made no sense. I asked him why had he done all these things. He responded you must give patients hope. "No," I almost screamed into the receiver but instead said with a restrained fury. "False hope is the most horrible thing you can do to a family. We came to you for honesty, for a second opinion and you told a fairy tale. Fred has suffered so much more pain because of your dishonesty."

The Long Story

WHEN I WAS IN HIGH school, I worked at a children's program during the summer. In the morning I would teach art and in the afternoon we would have free-play and then a field trip. Kids could play outside or sit in the air conditioning and watch a video or they could listen to me telling a story. I found it amazing at the time, but they invariably chose to hear a story. Perhaps you are picturing a few kindergarteners nestled up to my chair listening to a classic fairy-tale. The real situation consisted of me standing in a school cafeteria telling stories to 100 children from five to twelve years of age. Their sweaty bodies leaned this way and that as they sat on the cool mismatched linoleum and strained to hear each part of the tale. These were not just fairy stories. I told of history and comedy and even horror. They sat in rapt attention following every part of the tale, and as the story ended they begged to hear another. I was so happy that in the age of television children would still sit and prefer to hear a story. Looking back, I realize that re-watching The Muppet Movie couldn't hold a candle to a storyteller.

Stories are powerful things. Stories stick inside your mind and make you think. My husband Fred spoke often about the importance of story. (The last book I bought him was The Origin of Stories: Evolution, Cognition and Fiction by Brian Boyd. He was excited to try to read it, but only finished the introduction. He told me theory and Dilaudid do not mix well.) He was so excited by the theory of narration. I love to tell people that my husband wrote his dissertation on Buffy the Vampire Slayer. It always gets a great laugh. But few people know the title of his book. It was called The Long View: Three Levels of Narration in Buffy the Vampire Slayer. His thesis asserted that Buffy was filled with long stories. Each episode had a narrative arc. The season was a longer story, and the seven-year series contained an even longer narrative arc. Buffy the Vampire Slayer might have seemed like a monster of the week serial at first glance, but as the show progressed, a clear mythos developed and a plot arched throughout. On the surface you may believe this show was about vampires and demons, but within a fantastical structure it was really a treatise on life and death and endurance. This show depicted a reality where a computer nerd or a cheerleader could save the world. Pretty empowering stuff, don't you think?

Fred spent a lot of time working on his dissertation. He was very proud of it. Sadly, for many years I did not read it. There were plenty of reasons not to read it. It was really thick and complicated. I was busy with work and the kids. I had already watched the entire series with Fred and talked about it endlessly, so why read a technical document on the subject? And, in some ways, I resented it. I resented the years I had worked long hard hours at so many jobs while he finished his education. I resented the money spent and the life goals delayed that were part of the realization of this document.

No, I didn't read his dissertation, until he was dying. I remember that night well. Fred was still in rehab but he was failing fast and had agreed to enter hospice. I spent the night with him because I was so worried about his condition. I sat beside him and read his book. It took about five hours. At 3:00 am I finished. I looked over at him. His eyelids fluttered. He looked at me. "Honey," I whispered softly. "I just finished reading your dissertation. It is really good." He stared at me with a sense of resignation and disappointment and said, "That's nice." He then closed his eyes and resumed his slumber. I sat there numbly with silent tears streaming down my cheeks. I had waited too long. I hadn't read it when it mattered. I hadn't read it when it was symbol of accomplishment, a beacon of hope, the promise of a better future after years of hard work. I hadn't read it when it was a promise of great things to come. The book lay limply in my lap. It was a testament to what could have been.

Going To Hospice

FRED WAS TRANSFERRED TO INPATIENT hospice in Washington, DC, on May 20, 2009. The hospice was within walking distance from our home. (It was also in razor scooter distance, as I was the nerdy mom who regularly used a razor scooter to get around the city). Team Critical Care handled Fred's transport that day. They were so loving and caring. They were very concerned that Fred was failing so rapidly and called me on the evening of 20th just to voice their concerns. I was very touched by that. Of all the providers that we had dealt with in this long odyssey they were among the very few that ever called with their concerns.

When we arrived at hospice Fred was wheeled into his room. He was transferred to his bed and the staff asked me to step out while they took his history. I said no. I would not leave his side; I would stand in the corner but I would not leave. Then they began to ask him question after question that he could not answer. He pointed to me standing quietly with my three-inch-binder that contained all of the information about his prior two months of hospitalizations and said, "Ask her. She has it all written down. She can tell you." Then he closed his eyes. I answered all of their questions.

Soon the doctor came and spoke with me. He was a specialist in palliative care medicine and pain management. He told me that it was very likely Fred would experience a "hospice turn-around." Fred may be feeling much better in just 24 hours. He went on to tell me that the rehab had done a very poor job of controlling Fred's pain. The doctor put Fred back on his PCA pump and back on steroids to control the bone metastasis pain. The doctor was right! In 24 hours Fred could almost sit up. He could eat a burger and a milkshake and talk with his friends!

Fred loved to talk with his friends. He had a bright royal blue hospital gown he would often wear when they came. It made him feel less like a patient and more like a person. His fellow professors came by often; Michael Wenthe was a constant companion, but Jeff Middents and David Keplinger would stop by often as well. Both Mike and Jeff Middents had met Fred while he was well and continued that friendship into his sickness. David was a rare bird. He had never met Fred before visiting the hospital. He had just come along on a prior trip with Jeff Middents and enjoyed the conversations with Fred so much that he kept coming back.

Fred's hospice room was a swirl of film theory and semantics, as Fred would lecture like Socrates did while the hemlock flowed within his veins. Fred's mind was still sharp, although his body was failing him. He cherished his friends and their thoughtful conversations. In the last 12 weeks of his life, every dear friend and family member visited Fred. Both of his sisters had made the trip as did mine. His mother Joan was a daily companion and his father came every weekend. His childhood friends Alex Hicks and Greg Holtschneider had visited, as did too many school friends to name here. Greg had come all the way from his home in Missouri. Christofer Meissner, who was Fred's classmate from the University of Kansas, also flew in to spend time with him. The first person Fred ever spoke to on Facebook was Christofer. The last person Fred ever spoke to on Facebook would be Christofer. They were great friends, but so were the many others that graced Fred's comments field in the last days of his life. Fred's dear friend Jeff Miller, who had attended American University with Fred in the early 1990s and now lived in California, flew all the way to DC to visit him in hospice. They talked about horror movies. In high theory conversations I would usually excuse myself and leave Fred to his professor friends, but I loved horror almost as much as Jeff Miller did.

So Fred, Jeff and I talked about Abbott and Costello, Werewolves and Vampires, and of course we talked about zombies. We talked about the fact that zombies used to be slow. My husband Fred and I often debated this phenomenon. We had grown up with films like Romero's *Night of the Living Dead.* Zombies would stumble and walk slowly, groaning as they came. Even an out-of-shape store clerk like Shaun, *Shaun of the Dead*, could outrun a zombie. The terror aspect of zombies resided in their unstoppable nature. Zombies did not sleep, they did not stop, and they were everywhere. These are the type of zombies depicted in the 2006 book *World War Z* by Max Brooks. This book was a follow-up to the very popular *Zombie Survival Guide of* 2003.

The Zombie Survival Guide itself addressed a pop-culture meme of its time. In 1000 *The Worst-Case Scenario Survival Handbook* by Joshua Piven and David Borgenicht was published. In the series of books that followed the authors explained how to save one's life in extreme situations such as crocodile-infested waters or quicksand. In bars and at parties throughout America we took it a step further and asked all of our friends what was their zombie survival plan? In my age demographic, I have never met a person who did not have a zombie survival plan when asked to provide one.

Whilst this zeitgeist hobbled along, director Danny Boyle and screenwriter Alex Garland were creating *28 Days Later,* released in 2002. In *28 Days Later,* zombies ran. Purists will say the zombies in *28 Days Later* are only humans infected with a virus, but it opened the floodgates. From the *Dawn of the Dead* remake of 2004 to *Zombieland* of 2009, zombies now would sprint toward their victims, tearing them to shreds in seconds. I think this change in zombie behavior in media is a reflection of the culture of our times. This is only the most recent example of our continuing denial of the image of death within our culture. We can deal with a frantic moving creature trying desperately to live, but many cannot accept the vision of the slow decent towards death.

When I visited Fred's mother and father for the first time, I loved their charming home and was surprised to see a vestige of an older time within their walls. The Holliday house had a formal parlor. The parlor was furnished with imitation Chippendale pieces and matching lamps in a Victorian style. The space was usually dark and serene, a place apart from the busyness of the kitchen and other rooms. Once upon a time in America, everyone who had a decent-sized home would have had a formal parlor. This space had the best furnishings and art. It was the room where a sick family member would receive visitors, and it was the room in which the recently deceased would be laid out for presentation before a funeral. After the Civil War, families gave burying responsibilities to an outside business called a funeral parlor. With this change in the way Americans dealt with the transaction of death, formal parlors were replaced with "living rooms," and Americans began to distance themselves from the realities of death.

Another vestige of this time that is rarely seen today is postmortem photography. I vividly remember going through a tin of old photographs as a child. I remember holding up a picture of a "sleeping" baby and asking my mother who the child was. Even at six years of age, I can remember feeling something was not quite right within the image. My mother paused and then told me it was the dead sibling of my father. The child had not lived long enough to take a picture of it while living so they had a portrait taken after the child had died. I remember holding onto that picture for what seemed like an eternity. Although I placed it back in the tin decades ago, I can still see that baby in my mind.

When Fred met my extended family during our engagement, he held my hand as he patiently looked through years of family scrapbooks and photograph albums. After viewing a few albums, he was surprised and a little disgusted to see we took pictures of the dead. In our albums he saw my aunts and uncles and distant cousins all arrayed with their funeral finery. In 2001, one year before the fast zombie would make its debut in the world of film, I stood beside my husband as I took a picture of my dead father in his casket. Fred whispered in my ear, "Do not take a picture of me in my casket after I die."

A while ago I read Atul Gawande's piece in *The New Yorker*, "Letting Go: What should medicine do when it can't save your life." I was struck once again with the extreme discomfort most doctors have for discussions about end of life care with their patients. In our cancer journey, Fred and I often had to deal with the inability of Fred's doctors to talk about the reality of palliative care and hospice as an option. In the emotional roller-coaster of potential treatment and curative care, we were left without a very good understanding of the benefits of a palliative course. After Fred was no longer eating or drinking and was in extreme pain, this direction was suggested, and Fred signed the appropriate paperwork. When we transported Fred to the hospice facility, both the EMT transport team and myself thought he might only have days left to live.

Due to the excellent care of the hospice team, Fred rallied and he lived for almost another month. The curative care without a palliative component that Fred had been receiving at the rehab facility was killing him faster. I was therefore not surprised when I saw an Aug 19, 2010, article from The New England Journal of Medicine stating, "Among patients with metastatic non–small-cell lung cancer, early palliative care led to significant improvements in both quality of life and mood. As compared with patients receiving standard care, patients receiving early palliative care had less aggressive care at the end of life but longer survival."

So why do people resist the concept of hospice and palliative care when it has shown such ability to provide a better quality of life, and in so doing, perhaps even extend life? Why do all of those friends of mine have a well thought-out zombie survival plan but have never considered filling out an advance directive? Why do we resist the reality of death as a part of life?

I think we were cheated out of the few accessible images of death within our culture when zombies became fast. Death is rarely fast in the world of cancer. It can take years or weeks or days to die. I have talked to enough spouses and caregivers at this point to know the experience of death is often the same. In Dr. Gawande's article, Rich, the husband of Sara Monopoli, described her final hours. Rich recalled, "There was this awful groaning." There is no prettifying death. "Whether it was with inhaling or exhaling, I don't remember, but it was horrible, horrible, horrible to listen to." I know exactly how horrible those groaning breaths sound. I heard Fred make them for hours as he tried to breathe at the end of his life. But I heard them before in a pop culture world that tried to make sense of the senseless.

Hospice Cards

DO YOU KEEP ALL THE cards you receive? I do. When I have spare time I even paste them into scrapbooks in all their lovely glory. Behind each sentiment or floral cover, I cherish the words written by my friends. I especially love the ones from my late husband with his signature and phrase. He ended each missive to me with the symbols: "Alpha, Omega. Infinity." Which means: you are my everything and I will love you forever.

Those inside notes are priceless, but we should not forget the message that adorns each cover. Do you peer at your cards and ponder the thoughts of the individual that made each purchase? I do. You see my mother rarely writes more than a sentence in every card she sends. She does not think her words can say what she wishes to say. So she ponders each card until she finds the perfect one that matches her love of her daughter. She buys that one. She mails that one. I know to read the cover very carefully.

My mother depends on cards like the ones Hallmark makes to tell me how much she loves me. Due to the plethora of choice in the birthday card isle she always picks the perfect one. And so it goes for my son's births and other momentous events in my life. But in the summer 2009 Hallmark failed my mother. Hallmark failed my husband too. There were no hospice cards. For two months after Fred was hospitalized we received a tower of "Get Well Soon" cards. Fred rejoiced in each of these cards and they filled the hospital rooms, reminding Fred of all his friends who cared for him.

When we went to hospice, the cards stopped. We would get the occasional "Thinking of you" with the blank inside and few words from the sender. Or God forbid, we would get a "Sympathy" card. Fred raised his eyebrow with dark humor and would say: "I guess they don't realize I am not dead yet." Fred would still get some visitors and Fred would still get calls but I know he missed those cards and letters. It is very hard to die in the world of modern medicine. Patients are lost within a system based on curative models. Dying is considered failure rather than a natural conclusion in life. When a family makes the decision to go into to hospice care, many people just stop talking with you. There is a steep drop off in cards. What are people to do? Gone is the endless stream of "Get Well Soon!" cards inscribed with that most empowering of notes, "You can beat this!"

There are no hospice cards.

The mailbox is often empty, both online and in life. This is that quiet before the storm. The lonely solitude before the mailbox fills again with sympathy notes. Into this utter darkness a cursor would blink. While Fred was missing his letters, I was writing one.

The Onion Letter

My MOTHER-IN-LAW JOAN USED TO collect magazines. If you had visited her idyllic country home in western Maryland in the spring of 2009, you would have see them artfully arranged in crocks and antique half-barrels. They were quite pretty and colorful as a home accent, especially the covers of the periodical *Country Living*. I think she kept them all for some future day when she would have time do the projects listed therein. They were being saved for some better day. After her only son Fred died she soon got rid of them all. There would never be a better day. But in 2009 they were still there and I could still read them. Joan's magazines could be easily read and they spanned decades. Actually they were quite a resource, as I haven't found many of the articles from these periodicals available in a Google search.

I do not usually read magazines. I usually read books, online articles, or the local newspaper. I always try to bring a book with me to the beauty salon, as I find the pile of fashion and home care magazines a bizarre and foreign territory. Once I forgot to bring a book to a hair appointment and spent quite some time sifting through a shifting mountain of *Vogue* and *Good Housekeeping* in order to find one *Architectural Digest* at the bottom of the heap.

Although I do not often read these types of magazines, once in my life they were the only periodicals I read. In late March of 2009, I began reading these light and airy magazines as I sat with my mother-in-law at my husband Fred's side during his hospitalization. Most of the magazines belonged to Joan. She brought piles of them with her to the hospital. As we whiled the hours away waiting for a surgery that never came, we read. We read everything she brought. When we finished those magazines, Joan would stretch her legs and go to the cafeteria to get a coffee. Then she would stop by the gift shop and come back with another handful of magazines.

I find I hate most magazines published in March 2009. Be it *Family Circle*, or *People*, or any other title, I have read it cover to cover, and I loathe it. Joan and I would sit there waiting--for the doctors, for the tests, for some answers to our many questions with nothing to stop our frantic swirling thoughts. As we sat within a maelstrom of worry we read these magazines. Each night I would research kidney cancer online, and each day I would read about the life and times of Sally Field or learn the best method for cleaning a showerhead.

After weeks of such reading, Fred died in June. I found out I could no longer read a book. I could not fall into the warm embrace that literature had once provided me. My mind was a gnat always flitting away. I would prowl Joan's living room at 2:00 in the morning in the weeks after the funeral. Desperately, I looked for something to read. Under a pile of *Country Living* from 1993 was an old *Family Circle* with an article by an author named Ann Hood about onion letters and orchid letters. My mind stilled as I began to read.

Ann Hood wrote about her past experience as an airline attendant. She wrote about a concept called the onion letter and the orchid letter. Apparently, if a customer wrote a letter to the airline extolling her virtues and excellent service that letter would go in her employee file as an "orchid letter". If her service was abysmal, she might get a letter pointing out her many faults and that too would enter her permanent file as an "onion letter."

While Fred was in hospice, I wrote a very long onion letter to the first hospital Fred had been admitted to. This was the hospital that told me I could see his record after I paid 73 cents a page and waited 21 days. I sat next to my sleeping husband as he approached his death and calmly wrote a letter that referenced his medical record and provided dates and names and recounted the many types of harms this institution had inflicted upon Fred. My sweet Fred was lying there dying, and I was writing an onion letter.

Why do this? I wasn't preparing to sue the hospital. My reasons for writing were far closer to the reasons Ms. Hood gave for writing an onion letter in her article. I wanted to inform the management of this facility of the problems we had encountered. I had hoped we could encourage a necessary change within the organization. I hoped to channel the grief and frustration I was feeling into some kind of positive outcome. I also wished to regain our dignity, for in the process of becoming victims we had lost our personhood.

Fred was not the patient in room 6218. He was Fred Holliday II, PhD. I was not "Little Miss A-Type Personality". I was Regina Holliday. We had names; we were people. As I read Fred's record I grew angry that the story of his care never called him by name. He was only the patient, and I was only the wife. When did HIPAA compliance trump personhood? I thought of all the ways they took our names away. They dressed Fred in faded hospital gowns that made him look the same as every other patient they had ever treated. They made our friends and family wear visitors' passes every day. It was a nametag that called all of those who loved Fred a non-descript: "Visitor to RM 6218".

They wrote a response to my letter two months later. They said they would use my many comments as educational opportunities for staff. They had excuses for their behavior in virtually every instance. They did admit, upon reflection, that they regretted never having a family meeting with us and they said they would replace the broken television in the sixth floor waiting room. That being said, the hospital, the physician's board, and the insurer had decided that Fred had been treated within the "standard of care". Well, if Fred's care was standard, the standard must be changed. I would take our experience and paint it on walls and canvases and jackets. I would speak up. I would share our horror and in so doing we would slowly regain our personhood.

I went back to the first hospital on May 14th 2010 and told them of my advocacy. I encouraged them to place patient advocacy signs throughout the facility. Those signs would encourage patients and families to report problems with care received or abuse in hospital settings. The customer service representative took my name and number and email.

I am still awaiting a return call.

Ka-Tet

"I do not aim with my hand; he who aims with his hand has
forgotten the face of his father.
I aim with my eye.
I do not shoot with my hand; he who shoots with his hand has
forgotten the face of his father.
I shoot with my mind.
I do not kill with my gun; he who kills with his gun has forgotten
the face of his father.
I kill with my heart."

— STEPHEN KING *(THE GUNSLINGER)*

ON WEDNESDAY MAY 27, 2009, I met with a group of amazing people.
Christine Kraft had invited me to a small Health 2.0 meeting. It was an
informal gathering with no set agenda. Fred was in hospice and my life
was at a crossroads. Fred said I could come to this meeting and leave his
side for a few hours. He said it was a good idea to make new friends. I was
still a wife, a toy store clerk, and a hobby artist. In three days I would be
placing my first mural in the medical advocacy mural series. I met that
day a group of people who would support me as I entered a new life of an
artist and activist. In addition to Christine I met with Cindy Throop who
was working on health information technology policy, Susannah Fox

who was an Associate Director of research at the Pew Center, Claudio Luis Vera who was an information architect focused on open source, Nancy Shute was with US News and World Report, Dave Debrokart (by phone), and Ted Eytan, MD with Kaiser Permanente. I was invited to present a patient and caregiver view of hospitalization at this meeting.

I wore a nice skirt and blouse and was glad I did, for these were important and beautiful people. They sat large and at ease in their swivel chairs. I felt very small, and physically I was a good bit shorter than everyone in that room. I opened Fred's Dell Laptop computer that I had brought with me. It was a type of shield I could hide behind as I feverishly typed notes, hoping these people did not realize how out-of-place I felt. As Susannah began her lecture, I realized I knew her from the toy store. I knew Susannah as a really nice Mom who would shop for her children's toys without an edge of hurry or impatience. I knew her as a woman long of limb and filled with sunshine. I saw her walk within my store with a sun hat on her head and a smile upon her face. I would sell her toys, and she would buy them with gracious kindness and then depart.

That was my idea of Susannah Fox. I did not know her name. I did not know her job. I only knew that she was kind and was a good mother. This was a different Susannah. She spoke about her research depicted by colorful pie charts and graphs projected on the wall. She would list statistic after statistic about patient populations that were harvested from individual surveys. She would take all those individual stories and combine them and compress them into clean statistics or "hard" data. I sat patiently taking notes about the state of e-health and social media.

At around 3:15 I spoke. I described the horror of my husband being diagnosed with cancer and the terror of not being told what was going on. I spoke about the fight we had fought to get a copy of the medical record. I recounted the numerous times I had used the information in his record to improve his care. The record sat upon the table in its three-inch-binder. There was silence in the room. We were no longer speaking in the abstract about patients. They asked me to focus on what was the worst thing that had happened through this entire tragedy. I told them the worst thing we experienced was lack of access to my husband's data.

Within days this group of wonderful people would blog about our patient story. On May 30 at 4:30 in the morning, I would place the first mural called "The Medical Facts Mural" in Pumpernickel's Deli. Within days, the work would be shared on *The HealthCare Blog*. An advocacy movement was born. The "Medical Facts Mural" was a re-visioning of the face sheet mimicking in style and clarity the nutrition facts label: all-important, vital statistics were present with norms for comparison. How did a patient know if his or her blood pressure was high or hemoglobin low if they did not know what normal was? Where were areas of bone metastases and the soft tissue metastases? Where would you harm this patient just by touching him? Fred was injured twice by techs, who had no idea of the extent of his disease, moving his body. When I finished painting the mural at 8:00 AM Christine Kraft, Cindy Throop, Susannah Fox and Ted Eytan either visited the deli, took pictures or wrote about the painting in quick succession. I realized they had joined me on the path of the beam.

If you have read the Dark Tower series you are familiar with the concept of Ka. It is described as a controlling force in our lives. Call it destiny or fate, or even call it "God Moments." It is the energy that brings us together on the path of our life. My husband Fred loved this concept so much that his screen saver on his computer endlessly scrolled, "All things serve the Beam." Within the concept of Ka, exists the idea of Ka-tet. A Ka-tet it a group of individuals brought together by Ka. They walk same path of the beam towards the Dark Tower. They are one from many. In Stephen King's Dark Tower books his Ka-tet consisted of Roland- the

Gunslinger, Jake Chambers, Eddie Dean and Susannah Dean. They are on quest together. They are Ka-tet.

On May 27, 2009 I found my Ka-tet. Towering on the table my husband's medical record guided us. This was the story of Fred. Here began our journey. We would change the health system and create truly patient centered care. We would access the data silos that seemed too distant and inaccessible to patients and their caregivers. Since then, I have presented on stage many times with Ted, either on panels or and in a gritty TEDx duet entitled "The Embrace of Failure." We are great together. The energy of the other makes both of us better. When the patient and the doctor work together as a team great things can happen. Then there is Christine. She helped me in so many ways. She introduced me to e-patient Dave. She told me to get on twitter. She organized my first Health 2.0 meeting. She made my birthday cake, while Fred was dying. She came by hospice and talked with me. Susannah would encourage and advise me in the years to come. We were at MEDX together and she is in many of my paintings. She would also give donations to every rummage sale I held at the church in DC. Nancy Shute would write about my work, spreading the story to thousands. Claudio would explain concepts like open code so I could better understand. Cindy Throop would be a very dear friend who stood at my side and often visited in my first year of widowhood, even attending my son's school auction with me as my guest.

They were my Ka-tet and we were meant to be together. I had been well prepared to fight this fight, for I not forgotten the face of my father. I knew everything that had ever happened to me had steeled me for this fight.

Letting Go

INPATIENT HOSPICE WAS ONLY TEN blocks from our apartment and it was great to be so close to home again. I was able to split my time between being with Fred and dealing with the practicalities of life in the city. I even tried to start our car. It was covered in pollen and parking tickets. We had left in the same parking place for far too long. The engine rattled upon ignition. I went to my church nearby and asked Pastor Meredith if she could help me get the car over to the service station down the block. She said yes, and we managed to get it to the lot of the BP Gas Station at 5001 Connecticut Ave. The owner is a wonderful man named John Conner. He looked at the car and told me the transmission was shot and I was looking at about $1,500.00 in repairs. I began to cry. I explained we had just paid the car off, my husband was in hospice, and I did not drive. I said I was not working right now with Fred so sick and could not afford to pay 1,500.00 to fix the car. John told me I could leave it parked there. He said I should talk to my husband about next steps. He told me if we wanted to sell it, he would give us $100.00 for the car.

I did not want to bother Fred with the car. Fred was calm in hospice. It was serene and peaceful. The staff was very kind. They let Fred sleep and managed his pain so well. Joan and I loved the comfy lobby that we could rest in when Fred was talking with his friends from American University. Fred used his hospice turn-around well. He laughed with us, waxed poetic about pop-culture and prepared us for the fact he was leaving. Fred and I talked about the car and he made a list of things that must be done.

1. Get rid of the car. Get the title. Sell car.
2. Regina needs to get a drivers license
3. Pallbearers:
   David- Yes
   Michael-Yes
   Jeff- No
   Chris- Yes
   Greg- Yes
   Alex- Yes
   Jon- Yes
4. Plot in Grantsville is 20, 21, 22, 23 or 24 available?
5. Go see a movie every year on my birthday

I went back to the BP Service Station with the title to the car and sold it for $100.00. While there I told John about how badly Fred had been treated in many of his facilities. I said, "I notice you have a graffiti tag on your back wall facing CVS. I would like to paint a mural on that wall about my husband's medical journey. You would never get another graffiti tag, because taggers do not hit murals. What do you say?" John said yes. He said yes without ever seeing a design sketch. I would begin designing the painting *73 Cents* at Fred's side in hospice and I would revise it based on Fred's suggestions. Fred had been my artist collaborator for 16 years and often my harshest critic. He always expected the best work from me and *73 Cents* would be a masterwork.

Fred began working through his list of letting go. Fred was able to ask all his friends if they were willing to be pallbearers, only Jeff Miller would miss the funeral as he lived so far away. Fred Senior and Joan were able to get a plot right next to where they intended to be buried. They were concerned that there would not be enough room for me there. I smiled and told them not to worry. I told Fred many years ago in a poem that I did not want to be buried in a cemetery.

Saying goodbye to our sons was not on Fred's written list. That was too hard a task to write down. Our children were at a point of peace. They enjoyed playing on the hospice grounds and watching the turtles swim in the turtle pond. They would dance beside the fish in the fish-pond. They loved the toys in the corner of the hospice lobby, and they loved to visit Fred's room that felt like a home rather than a hospital. Fred would talk with Isaac and Freddie and tell them funny stories. There he would still do his finger games, like "here comes a spider" while Isaac squealed with glee. If you only had two minutes to say good-bye to your little sons, what would you say? What would you do? When Fred needed to say good-bye to his sons he said it with puppets.

Do you ever think about who teaches you how to die? Who teaches you how to advocate for those you love? If you are young and live within a peaceful land, you may have rarely experienced death. If reality has not taught us, then we can rely on fiction to do the job. Fiction and drama can teach us how to live, how to die, and how to say good-bye. Fred always loved to quote a line from *Grand Canyon,* "That's part of your problem, you haven't seen enough movies. All of life's riddles are answered in the movies." –Davis (Steve Martin) I couldn't agree more. I knew I was inspired to advocate for Fred in a hospital by watching per-formances by Shirley Maclaine and Sally Field. Who can forget *Terms of Endearment* or *Steel Magnolias?* Shirley's character advises every e-patient as she cries out, "It's past ten. My daughter is in pain. I don't understand why she has to have this pain. All she has to do is hold out until ten, and IT'S PAST TEN! My daughter is in pain, can't you understand that! GIVE MY DAUGHTER THE SHOT."

Did you know Fred Holliday, PhD., was a puppeteer? When he was in school many years ago he was under the direction of the Puppet Master

Gerald Snelson. Fred was part of traveling puppet show that would visit the local schools. Professor Snelson gave us what was one of our most treasured wedding gifts. He gave us the entire puppet set from his production of *Brave Little Tailor*. These are not small hand puppets. Think Jim Henson style puppets. They are amazing. Those puppets helped us get through many predicaments over the years. When we were still newlyweds we persuaded a few friends to entertain the crowds at Grantsville Days festivities using these puppets in a show of our creation. When our son Freddie was only 4-years-old he was invited to a birthday of his good friend Jack Taylor. Two days before the party I received a distress call from Jack's mother, Theresa Taylor. Her party entertainer had cancelled. Could I help? I had to work at the toy store. I couldn't help, but I said Fred could. Fred resurrected the puppets once again, and off he went to present a one-man puppet show before a room of active little boys. He was a hit.

For many years the puppets stayed in our closet as we worked so many hours at so many jobs. Then in spring of 2008, our family was at a crossroad. Fred was very tired and stressed. He felt he could no longer work long hours as an adjunct professor and video clerk. I was also very tired of working long hours away from him and the boys. So we came up with a plan. Two things could happen. In the fall of 2008, Fred could get a fulltime position at a college or we would take the puppets out and become a birthday party entertainment team. I would do the art projects with children and Fred would do puppet shows. In honor of this plan, I gave Fred a frog puppet for his 38th Birthday.

Fred was very proud of his new puppet. It sat upon the desk as a promise that life would get better. That summer the crossroad was reached and a future chosen. Fred was hired at American University. The frog puppet was put away, as we went down a different path. While Fred was in hospice he discussed with me how he would like to say good-bye to our boys. He would do it with a puppet story. The frog puppet would get only one performance. He told a funny story of the puppet frog sharing a story with his smaller frog puppet son. Fred had intended to do several puppet stories, but he was so sick in hospice time ran out. So there is only one good-bye. Fred was an amazing puppeteer; he could make you believe his hand was a puppet. But I am glad he had this chance to use the frog puppet, to walk the other path for a few minutes.

Our Final New Year's Resolution

AFTER A COUPLE WEEKS IN hospice the discharge nurse came to me. She said, "Your husband is stable now and we have to discharge him to home hospice." I replied, "How are we going to do that? We only have a one-bedroom apartment. It is not even handicapped accessible. We have two young children. One of the boys is only three and the ten-year-old has autism. So how are we going home?"

The discharge nurse replied, "Have you thought about moving?"

With only a few days notice that we would need to leave, I worked with our landlord to find an appropriate apartment and signed a one-year lease. Twenty friends helped us move to a two-bedroom apartment that was handicapped accessible. For the first time in our life Fred did not move his shrine of Stephen King books himself. Jeff Middents, David Keplinger and Michael Wenthe had that honor. We arrayed all of Fred's wonderful books around the living room in a type of formal parlor. The hospital bed was delivered, as was a bedside tray table. The oxygen was delivered next. Finally Fred came home on June 11, 2009. It was his 46th and final ambulance transport.

He would live for six more days.

At home, I was in charge of Fred's medical administration record. I worked with the nurse to fill in a pill tray with a week's worth of pills that would be taken on a hospital schedule. I was told that soon I would need to buy thickening powder for Fred's water. I was shown how to use the hospice "comfort kit" and was told to store it in the refrigerator. I questioned the hospice nurse about that. I pointed out that the box had a label saying, "KEEP OUT OF REACH OF CHILDREN." I asked how could we keep it out of reach if it was in the fridge? She told me the kit did not need refrigeration. They just told families to place it in the fridge because that was a uniform location that the hospice came team members had agreed upon. I replied that the comfort kit was going inside the hall closet on a high shelf in my house. We had a rambunctious three-year-old whose safety took precedence over uniformity.

When Fred came home to hospice care I had four industrial bedding chucks. One would be under him, one in the wash, one in the dryer and one ready to go. I would spend all day running down the hall to the laundry room and come back as quick as I could to take care of Fred's bedding changes. The nurse and I spent most of one of her visits just trying to do a bedding change. Fred worried so. He asked me, "Reggie, how do we keep doing this? I hurt so badly. I can barely roll over to help you." He hurt so much, yet he worried about me.

The hospice nurse was concerned that it might be too hard to take care of Fred in a home setting. She said we might need to go back to inpatient care. I whipped around with a steel glint in my eye and angrily whispered, "Hospice said we had to go home." She looked taken aback and stammered an explanation, "That is how insurance works. You go home to prove you cannot do it and then you can come back." I looked at her. I am sure my face must have been as scary as my father's at his worst, as I replied, "That is not how it works with me. You made us move. You made us sign a year lease on a more expensive apartment with no guarantee of future income. You uprooted our entire family in a time of great pain. I promised Fred he would never suffer the hurt of ambulance transport again. We will make this work."

For the last days of his life I sat at Fred's side. Joan often sat there too. She had been staying with us off and on for 12 weeks. She would leave every few weeks for a couple of days and try to rest, but would promptly come back to be with her son. She loved him fiercely and did not want him to go. As Fred grew more ill he would sleep and Joan would look at him and hold his hand. At night she would go lie down with the children, and I would sit alone with Fred. We would talk about so many things, and I would learn about the process that leads to death. I sat beside him as his hands fluttered and he plucked at his gown and blanket. His body had changed so much in these many weeks. His torso swelled, he was retaining water. I could no longer see his anklebones. Sitting up was hard, breathing was hard, but through it all he smiled at me.

Have you heard of the concept of terminal restlessness? When I first heard of it I thought of air travel and the endless pacing and waiting by the gate before embarking on the journey. But it has another meaning. When Fred was in his third week of hospitalization, we were well and truly into the realm of what often seemed pointless waiting. This was the week that the mad rush of guests slowed and time weighed heavily upon us. On one such day of waiting, I began to talk to Fred about Steven Spielberg's movie *The Terminal*. I sat at the foot of his bed and said, "Fred, I have been thinking about the movie *The Terminal*, and I don't think it is just about airports." He looked over to me at the foot of the bed; his too thin arms crossed upon his chest and managed to look professorial in a hospital gown. With his blue eyes dulled by morphine and pain he said, "Hmmm?"

"Well," I said, "I think Tom Hank's character has a terminal disease and he is stuck between worlds. He can't go back to his native land of the healthy, and he won't step out of the terminal to embrace a new and frightening place that he feels he does not belong in. So, he just waits... in the terminal. He can work in repetitive tasks, he can even grasp at love, but he is stuck waiting inside the terminal." Fred no longer looked at me. He stared at the ceiling. His chin slightly up-thrust and looking so very brave. He swallowed twice and I watched the muscles ripple across his unshaved throat. He coughed and clenched his jaws slightly before offering up a response, "It's a theory, I guess."

So, if I were ever asked what was the definition of terminal restlessness, I would have told you it was an apt description of a film staring Tom Hanks. After learning more about this term, I can confidently say my Fred suffered terminal restlessness, but at the time I thought my Fred was just being my Fred. You see sometimes before a person dies they go from being very docile and sleepy, to somewhat frantic and upset. They will try to get out of bed and walk around even if they have been mostly bedridden. They may yell or act as though there is something they must do, something they have forgotten. The term "Terminal Restlessness" makes me think of two things. I think of the term "nesting" as it applies to a pregnant mother. I remember vividly my nesting phase before the birth of both of our sons. I did so much on those days, feeling there were so many tasks I must do right away. I was pacing and doing until the point the contractions set in.

And I think of the night Fred died. I realized that Fred was suffering terminal restlessness. I fell in love with a man who paced, that frantically gestured, who liked to talk through the night about everything under the sun. Kidney cancer stole that man from me. Damn cancer for what it did to cause such a shining and exciting soul to close like a flower in the night. Damn cancer for taking the sparkle from eyes that used to gleam. But thank you to terminal restlessness, for the one night I had him back. For one night he was excited again. For one night he was frantic and anxious and exactly the man I married.

At 12:30 am on June 17, 2009, Fred woke up yelling out, "My catheter blew out." I called the hospice nurse. She placed a new catheter very smoothly. Fred complimented her saying, "You are very good at that." She chuckled and said she should be as she was a VA nurse for 20 years. She made sure Fred was comfortable and gave him some Atropine drops to help with lung secretions. Then she began to sweep our kitchen floor. I told her she did not need to sweep. She said, "Just go be with your husband." She tidied up a bit and left. Fred watched some repeats of Jon Stewart and Stephen Colbert, then he just wanted to talk. I sat right beside him, gently caressing his brow. We talked till dawn about our children and our life. About my art and our love of books by Stephen King. We talked about Doctor Who and so many wonderful things that happened in that past year. So what if everything he said that night didn't always make sense? He said it with passion. He held my hand with love and we talked until dawn. We pulled our last all-nighter. At 6:30 in the morning Fred turned to me and said, "Reggie you look so tired, you should go to sleep." I said, "I am tired. I will rest a bit." I slept for one hour. Then I got up to give Fred his 7:30 meds. Fred was very compliant and liked to take his meds right on time. I tried to wake him, but he would not wake up. So I crushed his pills and placed them on his tongue. Then I placed a straw in his mouth and told him all he had to do was suck. He did not open his eyes, but he managed to suck those pills down.

That morning two of Fred's friends came over: Jeff Middents and David Keplinger. Michael Wenthe had been by the day before. I warned them Fred was not too good today. I could not wake him. They came anyway. Jeff brought a book, *Lisey's Story*, for Fred. I laughed and said he already had it. He had everything by Stephen King. Everything. Then I showed them *Under the Dome*, the secret book: Fred's prized passion, his make-a-wish. Fred's breathing was so labored now. Each breath seemed like its own private war within his body. I stood beside him caressing his arm and holding the book. Soon it would be over. I ran and got the children from the other room. Joan stood on one side of Fred and the children and I stood on the other. Fred's hands were placed upon his taunt belly. He took a deep rattling breath. Tears ran down our cheeks as I said, "It is okay Daddy. We love you so much. It is okay to go." Then he stopped.

David and Jeff took little Isaac to the playground. Joan and Freddie went into the bedroom. I called the hospice nurse. She came and asked if I would like to help clean the body. I said yes. She said, "Please hold him up while I clean his back." Then I held Fred in my arms. For the first time in months I held him. For the last time in my life I held him. He was still warm, but he was gone. Then the undertakers came with the body bag and they took Fred away. When Isaac came back from the park his face was sticky from the ice cream that David and Jeff had purchased for him. He raced into the room to see Daddy. I told him, "Daddy is gone. They are getting him ready for the funeral." "Oh, no! They left his stuffed animals! He needs his bunny and his sheep," said Isaac sadly. The small menagerie of stuffed animals that Fred had received in the five facilities he was cared for still sat upon his night table beside his empty bed. I said, "It is okay Isaac. When we go to Daddy's coffin we will put them inside."

Then I went over to the computer and logged into Facebook and told the hundreds of friends who had followed our long journey that Fred had died. I packed a suitcase with suitably dark clothing and gathered up the children. Joan drove us back to Grantsville. At the funeral Fred and Joan stood beside the coffin and I stood further away. I did not mind. I had held him close till the end. Now his parents could stand at his side as all his childhood friends paid their final respects. Isaac placed the stuffed animals next to his father and Freddie did his best not to cry. At the grave site as Fred was lowered down, Isaac proudly said to his cousin Ellie, "My Daddy is in a treasure box." Then we went home to an empty house. We had a memorial service in DC on Sunday, June 21st. That night I posted a declaration on my blog:

The Battle begins...

I would like everyone to know that my wonderful husband, Frederick Allen Holliday II, died on Wednesday the 17th of Renal Cell Carcinoma. He was great. He was kind and caring. He was a loving father. He was a brilliant teacher. He did not deserve to die in such a cruel way. Cancer is a monstrous disease that eats you alive.

I cared for my husband for the last three months. My mother-in-law says that I am what kept him alive during his very long hospitalization. We spent three months in five different hospital settings. I saw some very good care and too often, very poor care. I found out things I had never wanted to know. I discovered how bad it can get when you are hospitalized in this country.

I did not ask to be handed this cup; I will drink from it, though.

I will let the anguish of us all pour out through me. I will be his voice. I will be your voice. We are all patients in the end. We should have the right to be treated with dignity and respect.

Up until now, we have only seen skirmishes. I have been waiting to begin the battle. Now I gird for battle. I am a liberal Democrat raised in Oklahoma by conservative Republicans. I am a Lutheran whose best friends represent many faiths. I am a mural artist in Washington, DC, and was Oklahoma State Champion in Original Oratory in 1990. I have worked in a factory, in food service, in retail, as a teacher, and served briefly in the US Navy. I am a mother of a special needs son and am the widow of a good man. I am the perfect storm.

My mother was a hospital housekeeper and my Aunt Minnie an ICU nurse. They always told me to go into medicine. Now, I will go after medicine.

I will stand up. I will not be silent. I will not give up the fight.

As a child, I was abused. I lived in a society where people looked the other way. My mother and my aunts did their best to help in a very bad situation. I went to teachers and told them the horror of my life at home. They did nothing. People saw me beaten in public and did nothing. Neighbors heard my screams. They did nothing. At 17 years old, I took my younger sister to a shelter. In so doing, I think I saved us all.

Today we live in a society that looks the other way. The health care system is abusive. People say "that's just the way it is" and we have to live with it. I say no. If there is a societal shift, things will change. Now if a child is beaten, it is not okay. If a teacher hears of an incident, by law the teacher must report it. I want the same awareness and laws in health care.

This week I will start my next mural. I will be painting at the BP Station by Politics & Prose. Look for me. Look for the change that will come. I ask for your help. Do battle with me. If we all work together we will effect great change.

Good Night and God Bless,
Regina Holliday

On Monday June 22, I went back to being an art teacher at our vacation Bible school at St. Paul's Lutheran Church. On Tuesday June 23rd I began to paint *73 Cents*.

Art As Medical Advocacy

The Cleaning of the Brush

They say that life defines art,
Or that art defines life.
I'll believe the latter,
Though others may confuse.

I've known art in my life
As others have known sight,
And have used it offhandedly
As others use their senses.
Sight is not appreciated
By those who've always seen.

As a child I felt it moving,
Outside cookie-cutter drawings.
Raw, magnificent, yet undefined,
It fluttered...impotent:
A bird without wings...
Until the brush.

Oh! I must have been a child,
And it must have been fun!

I must have used tempera,
But I really don't remember,
Not a thing,
But the brush.

To paint without fingers,
To carry out a line,
To a child what a wonder...
Who sees within the strokes: a form.

Yet, I was a child,
And though I felt the beauty,
I did not grasp the task;
For the brush was made of plastic,
To paint with poly-bristle,
Refrigerator art.

No. It wasn't the creation,
But the making of amends.
This set my soul on scaffolds
From whence masters dare to fly.
It is control that is seductive
The power of the god son...
Call it discipline or order
Or the cleaning of the brush.

My father was a man of his word,
And of his bottle;
Although sometimes one deluded the other.
But within my scant good memories,
Digs my father through a dumpster
To keep a promise to his girl.

Behind a school there was an artist,
Destroying his creations
And throwing out his tools,
Perhaps lackluster in his art.
My father dug through trash for
32 grimed paint brushes and a paint box.

He slaved for days to clean them
With sandpaper in hand,
With turpentine and soapy water,
Until they all came clean.
So what if bristles missing?
32 paint brushes and I still have some today.

But being young, my diligence
At cleaning was sporadic.
Oft I left my brushes
With paint dried in their hair,
Or soaked with soggy bristles,
And rusting metal parts.
Until I met the teacher
Of the scenic side of art.

She taught me how to clean them.
With her hands and soapy water,
'Till the water would run true.
She taught me how to mold them,
How to shape them and to dry them.
Think of bathing a newborn she said.

I continued in instruction
Still cleaning brushes as was taught.
Time passed, and I still painting

Looked up from my creation
To a man, my future husband,
Who in a year would call me wife.

I taught him the creation
As a Preacher talks of God,
And taught him absolution
Was the cleaning of the brush.

I guess we fell in love
While painting out our demons
On five by fives of canvas
That next week we'd cover up
Flirting at the deep sinks,
Cleaning out the brush.

I later met his parents,
And passed in depth inspection,
With my talent and our love,
With a great help from above;
And for teaching now his mother
The cleaning of the brush.

Some say the starving artist
Is a martyr for his cause.
That the master dies from slaving
On the ceilings of Church halls.

They dare to scream,
"He gave his eyes,
His ear and mind,
His life forfeit,
And died alone...
For naught but pretty pictures."

Yet, I respond defiant.
For in paint brush driven paths,
I met my husband, lived my life,
Wandered as a child in fright,
And felt the strokes that soften pain,
But not from any human hand.

Yes, I've known art in my life
And have accepted all night painting
With bleary eyes and tears,
But indeed without regret.

As I stare down at my hands
Hardened, chapped, and cracking,
I cannot help but thank the art
That tears at hands and heartstrings.
I cannot help but clean the brush
That adds value to my life.

~REGINA HOLLIDAY

I WROTE THAT POEM IN 1993 as wedding gift to my husband. I was too poor to give Fred anything other than my deepest self. I would remember that poem as I painted cinderblocks and bricks with the story of a life. When Fred was dying I wrote letters, poetry, and I would paint. I would pour my anguish into a palette and create the concepts that would soon appear on walls. Fred would look at my work with pride, but he would worry. "How will you manage when I am gone?" He would look at me. His face was drawn and gaunt, tinged yellow from cancer and failing kidneys. I told him I would be okay. I was going to change everything. Nothing would be as it was. "But, Regina," he said. "You are not very good at being alone." He was right. I wasn't good at being alone.

Loneliness had driven me close to the edge before. I told him, "Fred, I will not be alone. I have my friends, family, and God. I will speak for you and I will paint."

When I was in high school, I loved two subjects: Art and Speech & Debate. I tried to balance the two worlds and do both. I also felt the voice of God within my life and would attempt to present that message within my work. I wrote speeches with biblical references and my wonderful debate coach would admonish me saying, "Now Regina, you are writing a speech not a sermon, stick to the point." In art class, we were told to stay away from using religious imagery as it was considered controversial. In a defiant response, I chose to paint the hand of God as a tempera project studying the contrast of warm and cool colors. I was a good student, so other than the occasional rebellious inclusion of God within my art, I would keep them separated.

I would keep Art, Speech and God separated for the next 20 years. I could speak, I could paint, or I could talk about God's work within my life, but I could never do that within the same venue. When I began to speak after Fred's death, I would call it a mission and a calling. Many people accepted those words as secular terms, but others heard a deeper meaning. After high school, I would not give another speech for 18 years. I would work retail, I would teach, I would be a mother, but I would not be a speaker. Then in 2009 Fred grew sick, and I dusted off by brushes and my speaking skills. Fred died and I began to paint. I painted, blogged, and wrote speeches. I have never stopped. In a frenzy of creation, I didn't feel so lonely. God was with me and filled me with a sense of hope. I was in his arms. I was not alone.

So I ventured into the CVS parking lot with a massive ladder borrowed from my church, a pushcart loaded with paints and my brushes from my college scenic painting course with Fred. I painted as new widow still fresh in my grief. On the first day of painting Jamie Crausman came with the film team of Ben Crosbie and Tessa Moran. Ben and Tessa would film my work throughout that summer and create the film *73 Cents.* They were very kind. When I first began painting few people would talk to me. I was too strange a sight. People thought I should be home mourning rather than scaling a wall and painting out my grief for all the world to see.

I used a pushcart to transport large amounts of art supplies to the murals in Washington, DC.   Strangers on street or in the bus often treated me oddly. I would be wearing my old paint clothes and have buckets and brushes and bags of supplies. I would push my cart and say hi to folks. I would act the same way that I would if I were wearing a nice dress. I was being friendly and open, and it is amazing how many people would not look me in the eye. They would see my cart and swerve on the pavement. They marched quickly by and would focus their eyes far into the distance. I did not exist to them. If I had far to go, I loaded my over-full cart onto the bus. I would watch as a few passengers moved and sat several isles away. No one wanted to sit beside "the crazy cart lady." I'd quietly laugh to myself, but felt a touch of the despair and isolation that is part of the life of the homeless or strange. I guess it is not so surprising then, that the homeless people spoke with me first. They told me their stories in soft whispers and mutters and many of those stories started with a health care system that had failed them. Next neighborhood residents and shoppers at CVS would stop by my ladder and speak to me. They often had medical stories to share with me as well. As the summer wore on, I would paint in the gleaming sunlight. My ladder became a kind makeshift confessional on the sins of institutional care.

When I was a child, I knew sweat and thirst. In Oklahoma, a summer day would often be 100 degrees in the shade. My sister, my brother, and I would work for hours in the blistering heat; we would work either out in the vegetable garden or in my father's flea-market stall. We were dressed for the heat. We wore long-sleeved cotton shirts, wide brimmed hats, and work gloves. I would sweat so much that when I went inside for lunch the oil and sweat from my face could double as soap for my hands. (This was a good thing, as the restroom at the flea market often did not have soap to wash one's hands.) I was probably eight years old when I begged for water one day. My Father said I was just goofing off and told me to get back to work. I told him I felt shaky and dizzy. He threw me the garden hose. I did not want to drink that water. The water rushed out warm and musty from the hose. It tasted horrid, but I drank it. I was so thirsty.

I had not thought of those long ago thirsty days for many years, until I painted 73 Cents. Washington, DC temperature does not reach the highs of my Oklahoma youth, but it does get hot in July and August. One day I was painting on my high ladder 20 feet off the ground with no breeze and a temperature of 96 degrees. I began to feel shaky and dizzy, but I had to paint. There was no time to stop. I painted on, becoming ever weaker. I was interrupted in my painting by a voice below. "Hey Miss!" A lady called. "Hey, Miss! I brought you some Gatorade. It is much too hot today to paint without a drink." I climbed down carefully, my hands shaking as I descended. I smiled and thanked this stranger who was so kind. I chugged down the beverage and felt energy return to me so I could complete my task. I thanked her once again, and she handed me another Gatorade. "Here is another one, if you keep painting you are going to need it." After saying that she turned and walked away. I was so thankful as I returned to my painting vigil.

At first I worked in very short shifts. As the summer progressed and my painting shifts grew longer, I drank a lot of water. It wasn't long before I needed to use the restroom. Of course, I was not going to use a gas station bathroom. I have been in many service station bathrooms in my life and it has usually been a very unpleasant experience. John called me out on my prejudiced attitude. He asked, "Have you seen my bathroom?" I could not believe it. The bathroom in the BP Gas Station at 5001 Connecticut Ave. is beautiful. The fixtures and paneling are all made of stainless steel. The countertop is the deepest blue with specks and sparkles of gold. The floor is ceramic tile. In my experience it is always spotless. It looks like it should be in a fine hotel. John believes in treating his customers with greatest respect and it shows. I was so glad I was painting about my husband here at a Gas Station where people cared.

The Power Of The Suits

June 29, 2009, was a beautiful day. It was sunny and warm with a slight breeze. I wore my blue Easter dress, the one I wore at Fred's side in the first hospital, the blue dress I would soon wear within a monumental mural called 73 Cents. I was going to a seminar downtown to the JW Marriott in Washington, DC. I heard about this event through my friend ePatient Dave. When I wasn't painting, I was networking online and finding out how to advocate health policy change. Dave had spoken at the board meeting of National eHeath Collaborative on June 2. He brought my husband's 3-inch binder containing his medical record to the meeting as a visual example as to why patients and family caregivers need access to data. So I began to subscribe to the National eHealth Collaborative news feed. A few weeks later I received an invitation to attend NHIN (Nationwide Health Information Network) Connect 2009 seminar via the subscribers list. I discovered the world of free public federal meetings and I found out that most of them allow questions from the floor.

I had never been to a medical conference before. I had printed flimsy business cards on my home computer's printer. I went into the conference hotel. I could see an obvious divide within the attendees in the room, as I slowly descended the escalator into this new world. In groupings of three or four, I saw huddled men with long hair wearing polo shirts and talking with an isolated intensity. Or sitting singly or in pairs, were young men in hoodies with laptops in easy reach and smart phones in hand. On the other side of the room was a sea of men wearing black or navy business suits. They radiated wealth and power. Each man stood with commanding stance while conversing within loose groups. There were very few women. As I circled the perimeter of the room, I did not see the two distinct groups blend with each other.

I felt like a bright blue inconsequential bird in my Easter dress, as I fluttered among the forest of polo shirts, hoodies and business suits. Conference attendees in the world of medicine have a uniform look. You were welcomed if you wore a suit, tolerated if you wore a hoodie and ostracized in a church dress. I was not wearing the correct uniform, but I took a deep breath and introduced myself. I would say, "Hello, my name is Regina Holliday. I want to paint about healthcare to improve health policy for patients." I'd then say that I was inspired to paint by late husband who very recently died of kidney cancer. I would give them my slip of paper masquerading as business card. Then tell them to reach out to me via social media or email. Then I'd share the horrific things we had experienced during my husband's eleven-week hospitalization at five different facilities. I would see them step back from me with a brief condolence. A nervous half-laugh would often escape their lips. I was a widow fresh from the graveside asking questions that affect the lives of us all. I was not supposed to be there. They were having a ball and I was death walking among them.

The morning program began and everyone seated him or herself in the large hotel ballroom. David Blumenthal, National Coordinator for Health Information Technology gave the opening keynote. I listened closely and learned about HITECH and the term: "Meaningful Use." David finished his speech with the words: "I want to bring us back to what we are here for. We are here for the millions of patients whose lives can be improved by the work we do." Aneesh Chopra, Chief Technology Officer and Associate Director of Technology, was the next speaker. He spoke about the power of health information technology within medical care. Then he opened the floor to questions. A line formed near my aisle for Q&A. I jumped up and took a place in line. I listened to several complex questions before I heard Mr. Chopra say, "Last one, Vish, before we get hauled out of the room. Yes, ma'am?

I was at the microphone. I said, "Hi, my husband received his diagnosis of renal cell carcinoma on March 27. At that point, I began to email, do Internet research, try to find every resource I could to help him. I began to Facebook--Facebooked every night daily, stating his status, developed over 200 friends and then began to Twitter, ended up speaking to a doctor from Boston, Mass. Did everything I could as a caregiver to support my husband using the Internet. Developed a blog. Also asked for Internet data. Prior to this I did not often email, nor did I use a cell phone. During a three-month period I became complete caregiver and a walking PHR for my husband. I am asking you how will the patient and patient advocate be allowed to access the information of the EMR, to have that a standardized form, that we all as advocates of our spouses or loved ones, (can) provide the best level of data and catch all kinds of errors in the medical record?"

Thunderous applause filled the room. Mr. Chopra said that sadly technology in healthcare in no way matched the use of technology in retail stores. He added, "I applaud you for what you are doing with limited resources to try to help your family, but I am committed to making sure we have a foundation available so that clinicians on their own and by themselves and amongst themselves can start to have those kinds of transactions captured." Patient and family caregiver access to the electronic medical record was not mentioned in his response. I was determined to change that. I started to walk back to my seat when a man of the longish hair of the hoodie variety walked up to me and said I had to read the HITECH act. His name was Fred Trotter and he told me there was a sentence about patient access that we could focus on. We could ram patient access to the medical record through using that sentence if we really tried.

I thought about all of this as I left the hotel and went into the hot windy DC day. I descended on the escalator into the musty cool air of the metro tunnel right outside. My blue dress swirled around my legs in the uprush of air from the tracks below. There was ethereal music in the air as a transgender performer sang an aria on the train platform. June 29 was an important day in my twelfth day of widowhood. I learned about a sentence we could use to open a tidal wave of information. I learned the important people at medical conferences wear business suits. Soon I would realize that bricks walls are not the only surface you can paint on, but that is a story for another book.

73 Cents

*"I can tell you something about stories: they drive engagement.
What we typically don't consider (and this is why stories
are so controversial) is that stories become legitimatized
by their audience, not a storyteller. That is why some
stakeholders resist- they do not want to legitimize a story, a
rad idea or tribute or pain, by giving it a platform. Enter
the web, the blog, the phone, the community, the email
thread we are on. Stories. You know them when you
see them. And sometimes you need to see them to believe
them. This is the tribal vernacular; animal instinct."*

—CHRISTINE KRAFT

I PAINTED *73 CENTS* FROM June 23 until September 30, 2009. During that
time, each night I would promote the cause of patient data access on
Twitter, Facebook and my blog. On August 6, 2009, Dana Milbank
wrote about the painting in The Washington Post. He pointed out that
Fred died on the day that the healthcare reform debate began. The
Washington Post article had 485 comments and 358 Facebook shares. A
few years ago this would have been just a local story, but due to Internet
access it was spread throughout the nation within days. Most of the
comments were negative, but they taught me a valuable lesson. Working

with Cindy Throop we created a time line of my advocacy work to dispel the comments "that I was made-up, a fiction of the Democratic Party."

The painting became part of the national healthcare reform debate and was featured by the local FOX 5 news and the Washington, DC, NBC station, as well as the BBC (British Broadcasting Corporation), CNN, CBS, Voice of America, NPR, and the British Medical Journal. In addition, it appeared online at AOL, Yahoo, Salon, and numerous independent blogs. On Saturday, October 3, 2009, I woke up to find 60 messages and friend requests on my Facebook account. Three days before, reporter Andrea Stone had profiled my patients' rights advocacy on the AOL splash page. The *73 Cents* movement was growing and I had many new friends.

On the night of October 20, 2009, we sang songs to dedicate the *73 Cents* mural. The songs were from the *Buffy The Vampire Slayer* musical episode "Once More, with Feeling." There were over forty people in the CVS parking lot shining their flashlights at the mural singing those songs. There were parents from CCBC, Cub Scouts from Freddie's den, Fred's fellow professors, customers from the toy store, and students from Fred's class. Rob from Pumpernickel's was in the crowd as was my new friends from the world of patient advocacy. We wrapped up the dedication with the song "Where Do We Go From Here?" That night I said "That is my question for all of you: what do we do next? Thank you so much for coming tonight, thank you so much for being part of Fred's life and my life and spreading the word. And please go out tonight and Facebook and blog and post and tweet, and do not stop. Do not give up until we get change in this nation, until people get taken care of and we all have the right to see our own information."

Everyone had questions about the painting that night and wanted to know what each vignette meant. For those who knew my husband, they were well aware of his interest in *Buffy the Vampire Slayer.* He was steeped in the knowledge of the Buffy-verse and it was the focus of his dissertation. He said that *Buffy* dealt with death better than any other program on television. Other shows had their moments. There was the *Family Ties* special years ago. *M.A.S.H* and *The West Wing* each had episodes focused on death. But *Buffy* was steeped in death, and for a show that at first glance seemed bubbly and filled with pop-culture inanity; it gave us the most realistic picture of the condition. On every episode someone died, but they were the unknowns, the extras, the ones there just to die. *Buffy* took it farther than that. This show would kill your mother, your sister, and your lover. Just as in life, no main character was safe. Although sometimes they came back, and when they came back they were not quite right, as Stephen King would say. But when they died, and died without returning, it was as sad and final as it is in life. Fred often said there is no better media dealing with death then episode 5.16 of *Buffy* entitled: "The Body." Buffy discovers her mother Joyce dead on the sofa. Joyce's eyes are open and she lies awkwardly in death's embrace. This episode is all too real from its title to the massive sorrow of the grieving cast. Buffy did not stop there. Dark Willow was still to come.

In the sixth season of Buffy, Willow's lover, Tara dies due to a bullet meant for Buffy. Willow loses her Tara-her world. She is consumed by grief. In her great despair, she floats several feet above the ground. She has literally lost contact with the earth. Her clothing has become the black of the witch or the widow. Great and terrible she's become. Her vengeance knows no bounds and it consumes her. Only through the love of her friends is she able to reconnect with the living. Some of you might wonder what this has to do with health care. It really has quite a lot to do with it. Buffy was not afraid to talk about dying. Dying was part of life. What really matters is how we live while we are here, how we treat others, and how important it is to stand up for what is right, even if it is hard. Jeff Middents turned around in his pew at Fred's memorial service asked me, "Will you go Dark Willow?" I said I would. I suppose in a way I did. I floated above on my ladder with my red hair wind-whipped, painting a world of darkness. I lost my Tara.

73 Cents, my tribute painting to Fred, my treatise on the current medical system is 70 feet long and 17 feet wide. People ask me about the symbolism on a regular basis. The painting is a type of catechism that encourages the viewer to use the words of Martin Luther: "What does this mean?" The entire mural is framed in a stage curtain. Fred and I were both theatre majors when we met and this is our story on the national stage. The curtain is the red of blood lost in this fight for better care. Fred and I met while I was painting, and we parted as I painted. These are the strokes that soften pain.

Sheets of paper seem to hang from the fly space of the stage. They contain quotes to make us question. Quotes to make us think. Buffy is up there and so is Shakespeare. These quotes above are from many sources but all say the same thing. It is time to take a stand. Front and center on the mural is its name: *73 cents*. Coins are painted at the base of the image in this amount. This is how much you can pay per page for your medical record in hospitals in the state of Maryland. In Texas it is often a dollar. In Germany it was 88 cents. In the US, you also can easily wait to 21 days to get the entire record, but if the facility says they need an extension a family can wait 60 days. If the viewer steps back and looks at this painting, they will see it is large, painful and disturbing. No one is touching each other and all the figures are placed in darkness. No one is making eye contact in the frame. There is no communication. This is a closed data loop and the patient suffers.

Our family is at the center in this painting. My husband is positioned like Marat in David's *Death of Marat*. His eyes are closed and he is peaceful. Not quite dying yet, merely sleeping. He holds in his hand a paper that says, "Go after them, Regina." For that is what he told me to do. He said later that I should "pull a Regina," which means to go all out, never stop, and never give up. I am in the painting near Fred. I am the woman with three faces. A beautiful plastic mask faces my husband. This is one of those plastic Halloween masks we used to wear as children. These masks were a staple of my childhood. The flimsy plastic was molded in the shape of woman's face with too small holes for the eyes and nose. My face became so moist underneath as I tried to breathe while yelling, "Trick or treat?" These masks were cheap and well within the means of a poor girl. They did their job well; no one knew what I really looked like. Within the painting beneath the mask, unseen by all is my true face. There is only one photo taken of me during the first weeks of Fred's illness. I stand at Easter between my boys. I am terrifying. My face is white and monstrous. Fred saw that photo. Over all the many years we were together Fred saw me at my worst many times. I remember this one photo he took in 1996 while I painted all night on a dress-up truck. I looked horrible, so tired with no make-up and glasses askew. I wanted to tear it up. Fred said smiling "Don't, I think you look beautiful." Fred saw the Easter photo. He told me to destroy it. "That is not you; it is scary." Looking behind me my third face beseeches the nurse for information. This is the caregiver's face, sad and distraught, trying to provide help. My body pose is the same as one of the figures from Picasso's *Guernica.* My body appears twisted and seems to be straining to reach my husband, but cannot. It is as if invisible hands are pulling me away.

To the left of the family triangle, our three-year-old Isaac is playing with blocks. Those blocks spell out terms familiar in health care EMR, HITEC and ARRA. Isaac holds an "I" block. This stands for Isaac, as well as "Where do I fit within the system?" Isaac's eyes stare out at you like an innocent from an icon painting, questioning your soul, his half smile seems to judge your true intent. Above my husband, looking through the door crack is our elder son Freddie. His eye is scared and striking. He is distant and removed from the scene. Poor Freddie, he suffered so. An autism-spectrum child in a hospital setting suffers. All of the sounds and the smells assault his senses while the sorrow and fear assault his mind. I remember the day we told him Daddy had cancer. He sat in his visitor's chair nine feet from his father and began to cry. "No, not cancer, because I have seen those commercials on the TV. 'The race for the cure.' There is no cure for cancer, Daddy. You can't have cancer!" I remember the day Fred entered hospice and I had to explain to Freddie what hospice meant. He cried for hours and told me he was losing his "best friend." He told me, "Remember that movie we watched? The one in black and white, and then there was a flower with color?" "Yes," I said. "That was *Pleasantville.*" Freddie responded, "Disease is a lot like the flower in that movie. First it is just a flower, and soon the color is everywhere."

To little Freddie's left in the hallway a nurse is reclining in a chair drinking a soda and using Facebook. She is not engaged in the tragedy surrounding her. She is using social media but not in a way that helps patients. Above, within the room, is a clock with no hands. Time has stopped for us. Other families can go to soccer games, go out to dinner, visit a bookstore; our family is stuck within a moment even as the rest of the world keeps going. Beside the clock is the light from *Guernica,* now halogen instead of incandescent, as we enter a new age of technology. The fixture barely lights the few feet around it. Darkness surrounds the space. On top of the open door there is a large hornet.

When I showed my Health 2.0 friends the design sketch for *73 cents.* They asked about the hornet. They liked the picture, but the hornet did not make any sense. They recommended I leave it out of the final painting. I told my son Freddie about their recommendation that I remove the hornet. He was immediately upset. "NO, Mommy, NO! You could leave out everything else, but never the hornet." He looked at me with those striking blue eyes so like his father's and said, "That was the special day. The day you killed the hornet. The day you showed me everything would be okay. Isn't that what the picture is all about? When you see something is wrong, you do something to change it." So there is a hornet in the picture. Freddie was right. You could leave out anything else. The hornet meant everything.

To the right of my figure stands a nurse typing on a computer that is turned off. She appears to not be engaged, yet she is handing me an important paper behind the doctor's back. She is handing me the MAR or Medicine Administration Report. I need this document to make sure that the correct medicines will provided for my husband in the next hospital. Beside the nurse, the oncologist seems angry and not interested. A local child asked his Mom, as he looked at the mural, "Mommy, who is that evil man in the picture?" During the weeks I was painting the mural, several nurses came to see it and they still worked at the first hospital. A few nurses were amazed that I captured the angry expression of Fred's oncologist while changing his actual visage. Fred's oncologist is talking on a cell phone in the painting. He is engaged with technology, but is not using technology to provide care to his patient. At his feet stands a ram symbolizing sacrifice. The ram also looks upon the viewer but seems to channel the thoughts of the doctor. His countenance is malevolent. The computer stand appears to have branches that end in hands. The tree symbolizes the Tree of Knowledge. It is lifeless and its canopy is a blank computer screen. This symbolizes a circuit of knowledge that ends in nothingness.

Beside the oncologist and to the right is an emergency medical technician pushing an empty gurney. He is crying. His back is slumped in grief as well as in the physical task of pushing the gurney. He represents the 46 separate times we were loaded up and sent for radiation or facility transfer. Even though Fred's hip was broken in one gurney transport and he was dropped during another transport at the first facility, Fred came to look forward to the transports. For three to four minutes a day Fred could be outside, he could smell the grass, see the sun, and feel the wind upon his face. Between March 25, 2009 and June 17, 2009 Fred enjoyed about three hours of fresh air due to transport, at all other times this bed-ridden patient was imprisoned within a hospital or living room. The gurney points to a window in the mural. The window represents that freedom to enjoy life and to hope for a future.

The little girl America stands to his right and represents my childhood and our nation. This image came into the mural as the health care debates began and I saw kind, well-meaning people oppose health reform. I wondered, "How can you be against this?" Then I realized they were acting like people who have been abused. She is a pretty little girl with welts on her legs, and she is standing next to a switch. She clutches the caduceus. Most Americans equate this symbol with medicine, but it the staff of the Greek God of profit, thievery, and death. In using this symbol, I am pointing out that the little girl America is clutching that which is abusing her. She stares out at you with a sad face. It seems as if her eyes are asking, "Do you see what is happening to me? Can you make this right?"

Beside Little Girl America, we have a medical person tied up and standing in medical waste and red tape. This is to symbolize how the waste in the system is tying the doctors' hands behind their backs. I used actual pieces of medical waste from Fred' s room as models for this part of the painting. The woman looks out at us, her gaze impassive; she is just staring. She is neither despairing nor joyful. She is bureaucratic. To her left sits the waiting visitor. This man represents our real friend Michael Wenthe who kept coming back week after week. Very few people did this. He watched his friend from day one gradually fall deeper and deeper into sickness. He kept coming back. He went to five facilities and home hospice and he was there the day before Fred died. Note how far away he is from the patient. The medical process is distancing him just as much as the creeping shadow of death. Together, the visitor and medical provider are placed in front of an open window. It is light outside. There is hope outside that window. Outside in a stylized tree sits the blue bird of happiness. This is symbolic of the hope for the future, the love of the journey we had together, and the acknowledgment that happiness exists in the moment. The tree and bird combined remind the technology-versed of Twitter, and point out that hope exists when technology and patient care is combined.

To the left of my son Isaac is the housekeeper. I based her on my mom who was a hospital housekeeper at Bartlett Hospital in Sapulpa, Oklahoma for many years. She holds the tools of her profession. The soiled linen bag beside her is overflowing. The lack of staff in a lot of facilities has lead to trash and linens getting to this overflowing state. The sign at her feet refers to the slippery slope within the health care reform debate.

To her left is a physician holding a sign for reform. He wears a turban. He looks out at us with kind eyes. He is the other, the foreigner, who embraces reform as a right.

To his left are three figures at a desk. First we have "see no evil (insurance)." She is an angel/Roman god wearing a blindfold and carrying a blue cross and blue shield. She stands within a pool of money. Next is "hear no evil," a man representing small business with his hands over his ears and with a defeated posture. His desk is strewn with papers while time is running out. Finally we have "speak no evil," a pharmacist figure who talks into a phone with a mask over her mouth. Pills cascade to the ground around her feet.

To the far left a movie reel depicts the last frames of my husband's life. The film reel represents the media as well as my husband. The reel is in darkness; but if light is projected through it can guide our way. It will tell our story. In the months after the death of my husband Fred, I watched every video I could find of him. There were not very many as he was usually the cameraman. My favorite video was filmed at The Casselman Bridge State Park in Grantsville, Maryland, celebrating our engagement in 1993. It is 30 minutes of somewhat shaky video of Fred, his family and me. It is high summer and we were so in love. My favorite part of the video happens when the cap is placed on the lens of the camera. The tape goes dark. Fred forgot to turn the camera off and then placed it in the back seat of our car. You can hear the engine rev to life.

We drive away in companionable silence with only the occasional word being said. I remember we were holding hands; my memory recalls the details the camera could not. The sounds of traffic, the drone of the insects and a few quiet words fill the end of the tape. I am thankful for so many things as I live out my life. I am thankful for the love I have known. When I look at the final frames of the spool of Fred's life, I still can cherish companionable silence.

Impala Revisited

"1. Get rid of the car. Get the title. Sell car.
2. Regina needs to get a drivers license
3. Pal Bearers:
   David- Yes
   Michael-Yes
   Jeff- no
   Chris- Yes
   Greg- Yes
   Alex- Yes
   Jon- Yes
4. Plot in Grantsville
   20, 21, 22, 23 or 24 available?
5. Go see a movie every year on my birthday

THAT IS IT. THAT IS the list that Fred wrote. This is the to-do list of the dying. On March 31ˢᵗ of 2010, 2011, 2012, 2013, and 2014 Freddie, Isaac and I would go to the movies as would so many of Fred's friends. We would watch hundreds of films in honor of Fred. In 2013, well established in my career as an art activist and patient rights speaker, I would move with the boys to Grantsville, Maryland. There we could be near the boys' grandparents, Fred and Joan. We could live in the town that had embraced Fred when he was a boy. We could live near the final resting place Fred had chosen and place flowers on his grave.

Yet, I had still not completed all of Fred's last requests. I still could not drive. I had tried to pass the driving test many times in my life. I would get very nervous and would always fail. At the age of 41, I went back to take driver's education classes and would try to pass the test again. While taking classes Fred Sr. said we should look for an affordable car for my family. It would probably need to be a used car but it could be one with little wear and tear. There were not a lot of options on the lot the day I looked for a car. The best of the bunch was an Impala.

I wondered if I could drive an Impala; that car represented so much fear and sorrow. I got in it and I drove it and bought it. I tried to pass the driving test five times in my adult life. I passed on the sixth try. I cried large gasping sobs and held onto Joan when I learned I had passed the test. I had fulfilled all of Fred's last wishes. I had done my duty as his wife. This chapter was over and a new story was beginning.

The Writing on the Wall
By Regina Holliday

When I was only six years old, I drew upon the wall.
So sad, so small and all alone, I smote my cares on stone.
The other children swarmed and skipped
Like ants, they'd come and go.
I stood silent, chalk in hand and wrote upon the wall.
The teachers would pass me by and talk amongst themselves.
The children laughed and ran and played
And left me to myself. So, I would draw, and sculpt and scratch
The art would sooth my soul.
I left the best of me as powder on a wall.

At seven years, I learned that walls are hollow things.
That fathers beat and children greet
whips, with tears and screams

That gentle hearts can't help but bow before the rage.
Those walls give way to fists and boots,
while drywall cracks with age.
I wrote my sorrow on page and dropped it in the wall,
Hoping it would speak for me,
If I could speak no more.
Seven years old, I might be and slow and sad and small,
But even I could read the writing on the wall.

At seven years and thirty, I'd find the wall again.
I'd remember in my sorrow that bricks could be your friends.
That cinderblocks and stones can calm
That paint can make amends,
So, I painted all my grief out and smeared it on a wall,
And the children watched in wonder,
And a world would hear my song.
Sometimes within our sorrow, sometimes in grief and rage,
We can write our testament with gigabytes and paint.

When was only six years old, I drew upon the wall,
So sad, so small and all alone, I smote my cares on stone.
But I no longer paint alone.
For others hear the call.
Thank God each night my friends log on
And read the writing on my wall.

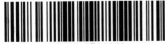

25667002R00149

Made in the USA
San Bernardino, CA
07 November 2015